F.I.T

Faith Inspired Transformation

Kim Dolan Leto

Editing by Layce Smith
Interior design by Layce Smith and Lauren Hall
Cover by Connie Gabbert
Photographs by Eva Simon

ISBN: 978-0-9907044-0-9
eISBN: 978-0-9907044-3-0

Printed in the United States of America

Library of Congress Control Number: 2014921040

First Edition 24 23 22 21 20 / 10 9 8 7 6 5 4 3 2

To my one and only Bill, the love of my life and my best friend. With all my heart I thank you for believing in me and pushing me to be my best. Without you, this book would not be.

To my daughter, Giavella. May you always see yourself through the Word and not the world and know that you are fearfully and wonderfully made and unconditionally loved.

To every woman who has struggled with her weight and body image: I pray the message in this book shows you there is another road to health and it's the only one that lasts.

CONTENTS

INTRODUCTION

Put on the new self, which is being renewed in knowledge after the image of its creator.

—Colossians 3:10 ESV

I tried to keep smiling under the glaring lights and cameras as the suspension built in the room. The anticipation was nerve-racking. Surrounded by twenty-something girls in the best shape of their lives, I wasn't sure I stood a chance at winning. The competition had been tough, and all of these women were extremely beautiful and talented.

It had been two and a half years since my father had suffered a stroke and I had begun my fitness journey. Perhaps becoming a fitness model and working my way toward entering the ESPN Fitness America competition was slight overkill. I mean, just losing the weight would have been a great reward, but something in me wanted to make up for lost time. Whatever the case, I had learned so much about what my body was capable of, and fitness had truly become my passion in the process.

Standing on that stage, a thirty-three-year-old woman who had painstakingly dedicated herself to losing weight and becoming an athlete for this competition—learning gymnastics, dance, and acquiring the strength and flexibility necessary to take on girls over a decade younger—I had never felt more powerful or accomplished. For this reason, it didn't matter if I won or not.

And then..."Kim Dolan Leto is our ESPN Fitness America Champion!"

It took me a moment to come out of my fog and make my way to the front of the stage. Winning was beyond my wildest dreams, but it quickly became a reality I was happy to accept. At this point in my life, fitness was everything. I worked hard to make my body good enough for magazine covers and fitness competitions, and now it seemed to be paying off.

My life leading up to modeling and competing looked similar to many other women's lives, which is unfortunate in some respects. For instance, I had a difficult childhood with alcoholism and abuse in my family and experienced self-image issues and insecurity in my teen years. Eventually I went to college and took the corporate job route in my twenties and thirties thinking becoming a successful businesswoman would make me happy. I struggled with my weight throughout it all and tried diet after diet into my adult years, but nothing ever seemed to keep the extra pounds off.

Even after I won the ESPN Fitness America competition, I struggled with a perpetual cycle of weight gain and loss. At this point, I began to travel down a very dangerous and unhealthy road of extreme dieting, and I found all of my self-worth in whether or not I made the cover of a publication or made it to the final round of a contest.

This lifestyle continued until I had a baby at age thirty-eight. Having my child so late in life made me reconsider my reasons for being fit, and I realized the methods by which I had been trying to maintain a certain look were not necessarily the ones that would ensure a long, healthy lifestyle. So, I started praying for God to intervene in the raging battle over my weight. I didn't want to have any idols in my life, and I especially didn't want my own body to be one. Turning to Him was my last resort, but it should have been the first place I went.

Ultimately, inviting God on my journey has been the game changer. He has shown me that staying healthy for my children and taking care of my body to avoid diseases that run in my family are better motivators than wanting to look good for a fleeting occasion. This is the answer to losing weight and keeping it off. And, in doing so, I have found that growing closer to God is an even greater reward than maintaining a certain weight. Focusing my healthy lifestyle on Him rather than on my body gives me the lasting motivation and the sufficient strength I need to continue on.

I wrote *F.I.T.* for the countless women who, like me, are tired of the short-term effects that come with fad diets. This book is not about working out for an hour a day in order to get a six-pack. It doesn't require you eat only 500 calories or avoid a certain type of food. There is no magic pill *F.I.T.* offers that will instantly make you drop thirty pounds. No, the goal of the Faith Inspired Transformation is to help women like you and me bring our bodies under our control and change our mindsets from temporary dieting to understanding good health as a godly lifestyle.

There are ten steps to *F.I.T.*, and each one will introduce various methods to help us stay spiritually, mentally, and physically fit. At the end of each step, there is a "Get F.I.T." section with a general overview of the information covered along with reflection questions and a number of strategies or charts that will help with daily application. *F.I.T.* may be read from cover to cover, or you may reference individual steps if you need help during any part of your health journey.

The 10 steps of *F.I.T.* are broken up as follows:

1. **Stop Dieting: Get Healthy For Good with God**—This is where we identify the failures of quick-fix dieting and agree to embark on the Faith Inspired Transformation.
2. **Renew Your Mind: See Yourself Through the Word and Not the World**—This is where we turn our focus from changing our bodies to changing our lifestyle according to God's Word.

3. **Commit to the F.I.T. Power Hour: Practice Spiritual, Mental, and Physical Fitness**—This is a daily commitment to spend time in the Word of God, time alone and in prayer, and time exercising.
4. **Dress Yourself with Strength: Make Your Arms Strong and Put on "Godfidence"**—This is where we learn about different forms of exercise and ask God to help us become physically strong from the inside out.
5. **Set F.A.I.T.H. Goals: Plan For Success**—These are faith-filled, accountable, inspirational, timely, and healthy goals and strategies we set for ourselves as we strive to get healthy, happy, and fit God's way.
6. **Eat God-made, Not Man-made Foods: Make Healthy Easy**—Here we learn simple ways to portion and enjoy healthful meals using the God-made Hand Chart and choosing God-made foods.
7. **Choose Self-Control: Find Lasting Motivation and Implement the 5 Ps**—By finding motivation that lasts (basing it in something relational, medical, or spiritual) and implementing the 5 Ps (Pause, Pray, Portion, Practice, Plan), we learn to practice self-control.
8. **Change Your Perspective: Find Joy in Every Situation**—In this step, we see changing our health and fitness as something we are able to do rather than something we have to do.
9. **Overcome Setbacks: Get a F.A.I.T.H. Lift**—Here we remember our F.A.I.T.H. goals to deal with setbacks and proactively strategize ways to keep exercising regularly and eating God-made foods even when our circumstances change.
10. **Celebrate Every Victory: Become a New You in Him**—Finally, we celebrate the work we have been doing and every victory we have encountered, no matter how small it may seem.

I believe you picked this book up for a reason, whether it be to lose weight, gain perspective, or experience God in a whole new way through health and fitness. And my prayer is that you will find encouragement and hope and the exact words you need to hear within the pages of this book. You have more potential and more strength and more beauty than you realize, and I think it's time to see it for yourself. So, let's get to work and become healthy, happy, and fit in Him.

Now all glory to God, who is able, through his mighty power at work within us, to accomplish infinitely more than we might ask or think.

—Ephesians 3:20 NLT

You have more potential and more strength and more beauty than you realize, and I think it's time to see it for yourself.

STEP ONE | STOP DIETING

Get Healthy for Good with God

Whatever you do, work heartily, as for the Lord and not for men….

—Colossians 3:23 ESV

Why is it so hard to make healthy living a habit? Armed with our greatest determination and countless diet and training plans, it should be easy; but many of us find that it's not. Somewhere between setting our goals and facing reality, we trade healthy habits for quick-fix gimmicks and temporary results. All the while our only motivation is too often found in pictures of actresses or models whom we want to emulate.

Growing up I dreamed of being on a magazine cover. My walls were plastered with pictures of models from the pages of *Glamour* and *Sports Illustrated*. I wanted to be like them, but it was clear to me that I couldn't compete. In comparison to these women, it seemed the list of what I wasn't far outweighed the list of what I was. I wasn't born with their build; they were taller and thinner, whereas I was much shorter and thicker. However, the images inspired me. So I began to place an unhealthy importance on my appearance and losing weight. And, by age thirteen, dieting became a regular part of my life.

Eventually, I became a cover model for health magazines such as *Fitness* and *Oxygen*. I achieved the thing I had dreamed of for so long, but I made mistakes along the way—the biggest mistake being my motivation for it all.

Since witnessing the effects a stroke had on my father, giving birth to my daughter, and inviting God to become the focus of my health and fitness journey, I have realized just how skewed my view was back then. Dieting was a means to an end—an end that left me feeling empty, exhausted, and ready to overindulge in all the foods I had missed and gain back every pound I had lost. It's clear to me now that the way I felt about myself needed to change before my body needed to change. But to get to that point, I had to stop dieting. Only then could I get healthy for good.

THE WORLD'S VIEW OF HEALTH

Let's be honest, we've all tried a quick-fix diet or two in hopes of "getting healthy." But often we find ourselves trapped in a vicious cycle of self-defeat. We question why we're not able to get *that* body on a magazine cover or television screen, and we feel defeated in our efforts to meet the same standard of perfection these images boast.

The media does an incredible job of showing us what beauty is *supposed* to look like, but the media doesn't always get the story right. From my own experience, those images we aspire to look like are impossible even for models or actresses to live up to. In reality, we're only seeing pieces of those women, on one day of their lives, captured at just the right moments, and then edited to perfection.

From photo shoots I've done, I know there is a strenuous process of preparation. I have to eat five to six small, healthy meals a day and never miss a workout for my body to be in peak physical condition, and I also have to go about my normal life leading up to the shoot: I still have to work, take care of my daughter, and keep my house in order. Therefore, I prep each week's worth of meals well in advance and get up early to train hard five days a week for the entire month prior.

On the day of the shoot there is a make-up artist, great lighting, and a photographer who directs poses and angles to produce the most flattering images. Once the best photo is selected, it's further perfected with editing software. By the time I see the final image, my initial thoughts are not, *Wow! I look so good!* I know better, so I think, *Wow! I wish I looked like that all the time. Photo editing is absolutely amazing.*

I am not offended by the photo-shopped images I see on magazines—I know how the process works. However, I don't want women to compare themselves to an inaccurate depiction of the way others look in everyday life. And while it's fun to dress up and take pictures that help sell products, I don't want to perpetuate any lies of an industry that might make women believe they are "less than."

Now, don't get me wrong. I'm not saying women shouldn't want to look their best or lose weight. However, just as I did, many women make an ideal look they want to achieve the basis for health and fitness; and, as we'll discuss further in Step 7, this is a motivation that cannot last. An even bigger problem is that the ideal look often comes with an ideal number on the scale and an ideal diet that will quickly get them there.

Consider these numbers:

- **"$20 billion**—The annual revenue of the U.S. weight-loss industry, including diet books, diet drugs, and weight-loss surgeries.
- **108 million**—The number of people on diets in the United States. Dieters typically make four to five attempts per year.
- **85 percent**—The percentage of female customers consuming weight-loss products and services.
- **1 Hour**—The amount of time spent in daily exercise by people who lost and kept off at least thirty pounds of excess weight for five years." [1]

You can't turn on the TV or open a magazine without seeing a dieting product. We are so inundated with infomercials and ads, but if these products work, where are the lasting results? If 20 billion dollars are being spent on diet aids, and 108 million of us use them, how is it that nearly 70 percent of adults are overweight or obese?[2] The answer is that we're trained in quick fixes that don't last.

QUICK-FIX FAILURES

My painful battle with losing weight and keeping it off led me to dark, desperate places where I tried diet pills and every fad diet I could find, and the end result was weight gain, frustration, and further self-loathing. Weighing myself daily, the number on the scale would determine my mood until God showed me how incredibly unhealthy this was and how to stop the vicious cycle.

Just as I did, I want to help you redefine yourself as a fearfully and wonderfully made woman of God and stop judging yourself according to the number you see on the scale both before and after you lose the weight. You and I are so much more than our bodies, and this transformational journey is about more than going down a jean size or two.

When I first made a commitment to get fit at age thirty, just after my father suffered a stroke, I was very unhealthy, overweight, and admittedly lazy. Making the right decisions about food and exercise seemed like a job. But, with a family history of heart disease, obesity, and cancer, I new I had to make a change. The desire was there, however, my understanding of health had not changed: I would still step on the scale after a week of eating right and exercising a little bit and expect it to tell me that I lost ten pounds.

Looking back on those days, I laugh at myself. I wanted something for nothing. I wanted results without change. I was hoping somehow, magically, I could do the bare minimum and get the best results. I tried every diet, and my weight would sometimes drop, but it always came back. I had to realize I wasn't the exception. I was just like everyone else, and health needed to become a lifestyle for me, not a race to get ready for bikini season.

There isn't a permanent answer in a temporary solution.

Dissatisfaction with our bodies and quick-fix promises make us easy prey to negative views of ourselves and the belief that "healthy" is only something we have to be until our weight-loss goals are met. We turn to quick-fix diets to lose weight, but when it doesn't immediately happen we quickly give up.

We see quick-fix makeovers on TV shows and infomercials, and we buy into the belief that the system can be cheated—that we can keep doing what we've done all along (maybe eating one less cookie here or there) and see drastic results instantly. On a regular basis my email is full of women asking if I can help them get a great bathing-suit body in two weeks. I understand this desperation because I've lived it, but I also know the reality of the work it takes to get that fit body. We can't undo ten years of not taking care of ourselves in two weeks. It's impossible and, on top of that, there's a difference between losing weight and getting healthy. The two may go hand in hand, but our first reason for losing weight should always be to get healthy, not lose weight.

Fad diets promise quick results, but they often leave out the education, exercise, and how-tos of maintaining those results once the program is over. And, let's be real, there's only one thing worse than restricting what you eat to lose weight, and that's gaining back every pound you lost. These so-called diets fuel the yo-yo cycle of weight loss and gain and only ask you to consider your outward appearance. What's worse, they make you rely on their product. Believe it or not, any effects aren't long lasting.

FIND BALANCE

People spend countless hours trying to find the "right plan" in magazines, Online articles, and diet books as if it's a secret hiding away in one of these mediums. But there are so many options and there is so much to consider. *Should I eat carbs or not? What is polyunsaturated fat and high fructose corn syrup? Are artificial sweeteners bad for my health? What does "paleo" even mean?* Between the varying opinions on what's healthy and what isn't, we are continually bombarded with the latest diet crazes, the newest schemes, and endless weight-loss supplements.

After thirteen years as a fitness expert, the truth I keep coming back to is that living a consistently healthy and balanced lifestyle is the only way to achieve and maintain weight loss. Personally, I don't like calorie counting, rigid diets, or any approach that feels restrictive. I find such methods to be overwhelming and confining. Additionally, we are all unique with varying tastes and body types, so we need the freedom to mix and match meals we enjoy without being locked into a diet simply because it promises to make us thinner. We weren't created to think about what we look like *all* the time anyway. Our motivation needs to run deeper than that. And, while it's undeniable that our happiness can be affected by how we look, we are so much more than our physical bodies. In order to achieve our health and happiness potential, we need to find balance.

With that said, I believe there's a constant struggle between what the world wants us to be and what God wants us to be. Extreme diets are a great example of how we allow ourselves to be defined by one limiting factor. We need to find balance amidst the chaos of dieting as we change our lifestyle and shrink our waist size. One of the ways in which we might do so is by changing the way we view food.

A New Way to View Food

F.I.T. eating is simple. Choose God-made foods instead of man-made foods. Picture the perimeter of the grocery store. This is where we find God-made foods—veggies, fruits, and meat—in comparison to the man-made, processed, boxed, and bagged food items that line the aisles.

F.I.T. eating is simple. Choose God-made food instead of man-made foods.

Our bodies need the right foods to function properly just as a car needs the right type of fuel to run. If you put unleaded gas into a diesel truck, chances are it won't go anywhere. Similarly, our foods need to nourish us, not just fill us up. Therefore, being selective in our grocery purchases and shopping only around the perimeter of the store ensures that the food we bring home will not be overly processed and will contain the vitamins and nutrients our bodies need.

Macronutrients are the major players in the world of nutrition. They consist of protein, carbohydrates, and fats (words I'm sure you're very familiar with), and many diets are based on altering macronutrient percentages or cutting out certain ones altogether. We will cover macronutrient balance and God-made meal plans more in Step 6; but, for now, it's important to note that completely cutting out any one of these key players, while it might bring results, may not bring us any closer to lasting health.

As we begin to consider what foods to eat, it's important to remember that God created food for nourishment, but also for enjoyment. Some diet programs require strict eating guidelines throughout the week and then offer a whole day off from eating healthfully, referring to this as a "free day," but this routine encourages participants to view healthy food as a punishment and unhealthy food as a reward. Therefore, dreaming of all the foods one might indulge in on their day off is counterproductive to one's health goals and can lead to an unhealthy emotional dependence on those foods.

To change our view of food, we need to recognize that wholesome does not mean restrictive or boring. God-made foods are plentiful, coming in a variety of flavors, textures, and colors. These natural colors indicate the health benefits associated with each type of God-made food.

Red foods: Cherries, pomegranates, red peppers, tomatoes, radishes, and raspberries all contain lycopene and protect against cancer and heart disease.

Purple/Blue Foods: Eggplant, blueberries, plums, grapes, turnips, and blackberries are great for your heart and cognitive health. They fight cancer and support healthy aging.

Green Foods: Broccoli, spinach, avocado, kiwi, kale, and melon support eye health, liver function, and wound healing.

Yellow/Orange Foods: Sweet potatoes, carrots, oranges, papaya, pineapple, and butternut squash support the immune system—protecting against some cancers, aiding in heart health, and contributing to good vision and healthy skin.

White Foods: Onions, garlic, bananas, mushrooms, pears, and cauliflower are beneficial for heart health, lowering the risk of some cancers, and easing inflammation.

Picture a man-made plate of food containing fried chicken, French fries, and a dinner roll. Some diets have a system that allows you to eat this meal and technically "stick with the program." However, everything on this plate is the same color, which means this meal is lacking the important vitamins and minerals that come from eating colorful, God-made foods. Don't limit yourself to a one-color plate of food. Experiment and enjoy the beautiful, colorful foods God made for you.

The Inner Struggle

If a house is divided against itself, that house cannot stand.

—Mark 3:25 NIV

When we severely restrict foods rather than simply choosing God-made over man-made, we set ourselves up for a vicious cycle of deprivation and overconsumption. Experiencing this firsthand, I learned how the deprivation-overconsumption cycle ultimately ends in weight gain.

When I first began dieting at age thirteen, I tried to severely restrict the amount of carbohydrates I consumed, but it backfired on me. I did pretty well for a few days, and then I was so hungry that I found myself dreaming about pizza. I could only hold out for so long before indulging—eating way too much. My food guilt led me to the scale, and I vowed to go back on my diet when I saw the number, which led to another diet and another and another and so on.

The vicious cycles associated with diets can repeat themselves until we educate ourselves and tackle the root of the issue (more on this in Step 2). We can only endure deprivation for so long before our pre-diet habits kick back in. After that, we tend to overindulge in all of our favorite "cheat" foods because we feel we deserve them or because our bodies think they hold the sustenance we need after essentially starving ourselves, and this often causes the weight gain.

Many of us can't get off of the roller coaster of weight gain and loss because dieting disrupts our internal balance. Focusing on counting calories or avoiding certain foods—tasks that make us feel limited—distracts us from enjoying foods we *can* eat and experimenting with new, creative options that seem unlimited. In short, focusing on what we can't have makes us want it that much more and causes us to war against ourselves. This often leads to unhealthy inner dialogue.

I'm embarrassed to admit the self-berating talk that used to go on in my mind. Even in the middle of the night I would wake up and think about everything I ate the day before. If it was a day I splurged, I felt bad about myself and promised to be better the next day. Always the fear of failure was present, and the internal struggle between feeling I had worked hard and deserved food and feeling I was still lacking and should give up was maddening at times.

Consider the words you say to/about yourself:

- Do your words encourage and affirm your goals?
- Do you refer to yourself in parts—negatively focusing on your thighs or arms or stomach?
- Do you talk failure and expect success?
- Do you build yourself up or tear yourself down on a regular basis?

Your body hears and is deeply affected by everything you say. We're physical, emotional, and spiritual beings, so all three aspects of us need to be committed to the same mission. We need to make sure that the words we say and the foods we choose to eat align with our goals in order to find peace and balance and avoid inner turmoil.

Spirit vs. Flesh

If any of you lacks wisdom, you should ask God, who gives generously to all without finding fault, and it will be given to you.

—James 1:5 NIV

I used to pray, "God, please help me. I need more of you," but I realized God was saying, "I'm here. You already have all of me, but do I have all of you?"

When we walk with God and pursue things of Him, we feed our spirit and it gets stronger. But when we walk in the flesh, our spirit is malnourished and weak. The flesh continually makes the same disappointing decisions and leaves us feeling powerless. It's driven by emotions, and it doesn't care what we really want because it wants what it wants and it wants it now.

One day at Target, my three-year-old was begging me for a toy. I watched my sweet, normally well-behaved child throw herself on the floor, kicking and screaming. She was throwing a fit, and I knew it was a defining moment for us. There wasn't any room in the aisle as the scene continued, so I actually had to step over her. When I did that, she stopped crying and our eyes met. She was ready to lock horns with me, but she knew I wasn't changing my mind. So, she got off the floor, and that was it.

Sometimes our flesh is just like my three-year-old daughter throwing a fit in the middle of Target. It doesn't consider the outcome of its behavior, and it doesn't care why the answer is what it is. It only cares about indulging itself in the moment.

When I was a new Christian, I remember hearing my pastor talk about the flesh warring against the spirit, but I had no idea what he meant. As I have walked farther with God and grown closer to Him, I now see the ways in which my flesh bosses me around. However, my walk with God has also taught me that, through Him, I am able to overcome the tantrums of the flesh, and so are you.

The Spirit of God enables us to practice self-control whenever our flesh is screaming for a chocolate chip cookie. Let's be honest, most of us have had plenty of cookies won by our inconsolable flesh, but when we listen to that still, small voice, we have power—power and the ability to say yes to who we really want to be and to make the decisions we really want to make.

> **But I say, walk by the Spirit, and you will not gratify the desires of the flesh. For the desires of the flesh are against the Spirit, and the desires of the Spirit are against the flesh, for these are opposed to each other, to keep you from doing the things you want to do.**
>
> **—Galatians 5:16-17 ESV**

Like finances, marriage, and other subjects studied through the Word in our churches, a healthy approach to life can be attained when our focus is on God. We can't get healthy, remain balanced, and maintain the results on our strength alone because healthy is so much more than a look we are trying to obtain; it's a lifestyle we are trying to maintain.

Healthy is so much more than a look we are trying to obtain; it's a lifestyle we are trying to maintain.

Changing the way we eat or the amount of time we exercise will bring results, but those results won't last if there is nothing to sustain us. God's Word says if we walk by the Spirit, then we will overcome our flesh. But how do we do that?

> **The Lord directs the steps of the godly. He delights in every detail of their lives. Though they stumble, they will never fall, for the Lord holds them by the hand.**
>
> **—Psalm 37:23-24 NLT**

Connecting to God through prayer and His Word is the way we overcome our flesh in order to take the next steps in our Faith Inspired Transformation. Diets are not the answer; changing how we view our food and ourselves is. Think about what you eat on a regular basis (even if you are on a strict diet) and determine if it's bringing balance or causing more chaos in your life.

Throughout the day, think about what you can eat, not what you can't. For example, every day I try to fit a salad, nuts, yogurt, Ezekiel bread, a couple servings of fruit, some steamed veggies, and lean protein into my meals. Focusing on what I can eat instead of what I can't or shouldn't helps me make good decisions when buying and preparing food. I'm not tempted by anything unhealthy because I haven't made that an option.

Whenever you sit down for a meal, look at your plate. Is it filled with colors? Is your food natural, or did it come from a bag or box? Don't let all the varying opinions confuse you. Focus on what you can eat, and stop relying on dieting programs that only cause more imbalances as the flesh wars against the spirit.

Dear friend, I pray that you may enjoy good health and that all may go well with you, even as your soul is getting along well.

—3 John 1:2 NIV

When we're seeking Him along this journey, we achieve health the right way—from the inside out. Combining our faith with fitness may seem like a new concept for some, but how good are we for God when we feel overweight, tired, and depressed about the way we look?

As Christians, we often give ourselves a pass because we think taking care of ourselves is vain, but we shouldn't confuse vanity with health. Keeping our focus on Him and seeking a healthy lifestyle with Him is the answer. There is no vanity in that. It's a life I believe God wants to give us, and the results of such a life are eternal and never fleeting.

GOD GIVES US OUR DESIRES

If you, then, though you are evil, know how to give good gifts to your children, how much more will your Father in heaven give good gifts to those who ask him!
—Matthew 7:11 NIV

Becoming a mother showed me a type of love I had never known before. As the oldest of five kids (and spending way too much time as the babysitter), I never thought I would have my own children. I gained my husband's two boys, whom I adore and love as my own, when we got married, and I thought that was it for me having children. However, after five years of being married, a causal conversation one warm, summer night changed everything. On this night my husband and I were sitting in our backyard talking when he suddenly looked at me and said, "If you died tonight, what would you regret?

This was a difficult question for me to answer honestly because I had been feeling that pull on my heart to have a baby. When I told him, "I would regret that we never had a child," he agreed.

I knew God had spoken to both of us and changed our hearts and minds, and being pregnant was one of the happiest times of my life. The love I felt for my daughter when she was born was the purest and most selfless love I had ever experienced, so when I read the scripture above, it's hard for me to fathom that God loves me (and you) so much more.

Think about how much you love your children. Consider all the time and energy you put into making sure they have everything they need. Think of all the little, daily tasks you perform for your children: cooking, driving, cleaning, helping with school projects, tucking them into bed at night—this list is endless and lovingly selfless.

Now, since you would do something as detailed and thoughtful as making sure your child doesn't go to sleep without being told they are loved, become confidently aware that God wants to do even more for you. Let this sink in and fill you with faith. When this realization comes over me, I have no choice but to feel bold and strong in Him.

God places desires in our hearts that will lead us to the best life we can possibly live in Him. Your health should be important to you because it's important to God. Don't you think he wants you to enjoy a long, healthy life? Don't you think he wants you to play with your grandchildren someday? He's willing to do his part to get you there. Are you willing to do yours?

Start Now

> **For I am about to do something new. See, I have already begun! Do you not see it? I will make a pathway through the wilderness. I will create rivers in the dry wasteland.**
>
> **—Isaiah 43:19 NLT**

Have you ever considered how much your health affects your daily life?

- **How many clothes are hanging in your closet right now that you plan on wearing someday?**
- **Does getting dressed stress you out?**
- **When you have to go to a party, does thinking about what you're going to wear make you want to stay home?**
- **When you look in the mirror, are you happy with what you see?**
- **Do you feel tired all the time?**
- **Do you avoid and fear running into people from your past?**
- **Do you look forward to indulging in comfort foods and then feel bad for eating them?**
- **Are you sick of dieting?**

Do you think your heavenly father wants you fretting over issues that steal your time away from the blessed life he wants to walk you through?

You don't have to feel this way. Right now you are good enough in God. More importantly, He wants to free you from the bondage of restrictive diets and an unhealthy lifestyle. Do you have faith that God will do a new thing in your life?

It's time to become a new you in Him. It's never too late to get started. Don't let the fear of failure rob you of the desire to change, and never discount even the smallest victory. But don't try to change your lifestyle by your own strength either. Even the strongest will eventually need help. Don't waste the work God has done and wants to continue in your life.

Yes, you have it in you! Love yourself enough to break free from dieting. Rely on God's power, not will power, and trade temporary fixes for a healthy and permanent Faith Inspired Transformation. So, start now, follow the principles in this book, pray for guidance, and give each day your best.

Change is the answer. Faith is the fuel. And discipline is the vehicle to take you there.

Fight the good fight for the true faith. Hold tightly to the eternal life to which God has called you, which you have confessed so well before many witnesses.

—1 Timothy 6:12 NLT

GET F.I.T.

Step one of our Faith Inspired Transformation helps us to understand that healthy goals don't have a finish line—only diets do. We're not on a diet; we're making health our lifestyle by transforming ourselves through faith in God one day at a time. Here we commit to stop dieting and to start getting healthy with God-made foods.

Reflection Questions:

- What diets have you tried in the past? Were the results lasting?

  ____

  ____

  ____

- Do you think your efforts to lose weight have been God-honoring in the past? How do you hope to change your approach?

  ____

  ____

  ____

By seeking God on this journey through prayer and scripture, we get off the roller coaster of yo-yo dieting and get ready to take the next step toward renewing our minds. It takes twenty-one days to form a habit, so do your best to implement the following strategies for that amount of time.

Strategy #1: Ask God to help you control your appetite before every meal.

Strategy #2: Take the first step in shifting your focus from the world to the Word: choose scripture over social media, television, or a magazine at least once each day.

Strategy #3: Practice accepting yourself the way you are now. Look in the mirror every day and find one new thing you like about yourself.

Strategy #4: Immediately replace any negative thoughts or words about your appearance or health with positive ones.

Strategy #5: Find balance every day by making healthy eating decisions, doing some form of exercise, and thinking positively.

STEP TWO | RENEW YOUR MIND

See Yourself Through the Word, Not the World

For as he thinks within himself, so he is.
—Proverbs 23:7 NASB

Standing in my kitchen at Christmastime, my 60-year-old mother was explaining to me how she could never again be the same size she was in high school. As she listed her reasons why it was impossible, I stopped her and said, "You're right. You can't because you've set that limit on yourself. The Bible says we can't be any better than we think: 'As a man thinks, so is he.'"

My mom loves the Lord, and she was shocked when she realized she could go to Him with such concerns in her life. A few weeks later, she excitedly pulled a piece of folded paper out of her pocket and handed it to me. It was an entrance form to a triathlon, and she was beaming. She signed up, and it was exactly the time-based goal she needed. The triathlon training made her focused and committed to biking, swimming, and running, and her new mindset empowered her to make the right food choices. If she didn't renew her mind and put the date on the calendar, I bet she would still be talking about losing weight instead of doing it.

Now, three years later and with two triathlons under her belt, my mother is the same size she was in high school. She is healthier and happier than ever, and everything about her has changed from the inside out. Even after my father passed away between her two triathlons, she didn't give up. Armed with the Word, she takes one workout and meal at a time and keeps transforming herself through faith in Him.

Don't put limitations on yourself the way my mother once did, the way so many of us do. Don't say to yourself…

I could never be that size again.

I've had children—my body is ruined.

I'm too old, and it's too late.

God desires health for us, and He reminds us again and again through scripture that He wants to give us the desires of our hearts, that He desires good things for us, and that all we need to do is seek Him first and all of these desires and good things will be added to our lives.

IDENTIFY NEGATIVE THOUGHTS

If we become our thoughts, our thoughts design our future. Our thoughts dictate our actions: if you believe you can't do something, you can't. This can work for or against us, so let's take a look at the little voices that talk to us all day long.

Don't let your "inner me" become your enemy. Whatever you're going through stops controlling you today.

Our experiences—pivotal moments from childhood, things we've heard others say about themselves, things others have said about us, the good and bad gained from our relationships—design our inner voices and act as the filters through which we see life. Any time we're exposed to new situations, our minds search through internal databases and assume responses based on these cumulative experiences.

Our minds are like tape recorders. They store every word we say to ourselves and play them back to us over and over again. Therefore, it's vital that we speak God's truth. When we speak His positive words over ourselves, we plant the seeds of success because what we think about is what we become.

I struggled so long with insecurity about my weight and often wondered where it came from. After spending some time sifting through my past, I remembered my mom telling me I looked fat on my first day of eighth grade. Now, I don't think my mom meant to hurt me, but her words stayed with me all the same. They changed how I saw myself so that, at thirteen, what I weighed and how I looked took on new importance. I felt myself turn inward. I felt ugly, ashamed, and really hurt. My self-esteem was shattered, and I never confronted the pain.

Can you think of anything hurtful someone has said that you've never dealt with? Perhaps your ex-boyfriend told you he preferred blonde hair to your brunette mane, or your family let it be known that you were the less attractive sister, or maybe in high school people called you ugly or fat. Do some deep soul-searching and pinpoint these moments. Once you know where your hurt began, forgive the person or the people who said it.

We may think people don't always deserve our forgiveness, but forgiveness is really a gift we give ourselves. Other people hold power over us and we distance ourselves from the blessings of God when we withhold forgiveness and cling to a grudge. I don't know about you, but I don't want anything to keep me from the blessings God provides in this life.

> **I tell you, you can pray for anything, and if you believe that you've received it, it will be yours. But when you are praying, first forgive anyone you are holding a grudge against, so that your Father in heaven will forgive your sins, too.**
>
> **—Mark 11:24-25 NLT**

Comments from people can really affect how we see ourselves. However, it's important to remember that just because someone says something doesn't make it true. People speak from their own limitations, so if they don't think something is possible for them, it must be impossible for everyone. If God put a dream in your heart, don't let other people deceive you. Finally understanding what caused my negative self-talk enabled me to find healing and believe in my ability to get healthy for good, and it can be the turning point for you too.

BRING IT TO LIGHT

I pray that out of his glorious riches he may strengthen you with power through his Spirit in your inner being.

—Ephesians 3:16 NIV

At some point in your life (maybe now), certain memories or experiences have held you back. A barrier was created, and you couldn't move past it. But God doesn't want that; He wants us to live in freedom. There is nothing you've done that God won't forgive, forget, heal, or change. Nothing in your past should be hindering your future.

Depression, anxiety, and stress become issues in our lives when pain goes unaddressed. I've learned that things are so much bigger and more powerful when they are hidden and not dealt with. But, when we talk about the pain we feel from the lies we believe, those things that have kept us in darkness begin to dissipate because bringing our issues to light opens the door to truth.

We need to remember that God is real and He cares about all the details of our lives. God wants things to go well for us. We're not supposed to struggle in our own strength, but there is an enemy who wants to keep us in the dark—believing we cannot be happy, thinking we must fit one definition of beauty, and keeping God separate from our health and fitness goals. As we journey on toward the renewal of our minds and bodies, understanding our thoughts and remembering who God says we are will be our greatest weapons against the lies that come our way.

IDENTIFY NEGATIVE PATTERNS

Whether you think you can or you think you can't—you're right.

—Henry Ford

You can only go as far as your thinking will take you, and in order to become a new you, the old you must go. Sometimes this is difficult, but would you rather have the pain of change or the pain of staying the same? Remaining stagnant can lead to or continue to foster unhappiness. But change, while sometimes uncomfortable, will bring growth.

Would you rather have the pain of change or the pain of staying the same?

A good friend of mine hated, and I mean absolutely detested her job. She was miserable every time I spoke to her—rattling off a list of unending complaints: her boss was demanding, her hours were ridiculous, and her pay was meager. The answer seemed obvious (get a new job), but she stayed. One day I finally told her she was living in her own prison and only she had the keys to get out. She was dead silent and then suddenly declared that she was going to look for a new job.

You might feel trapped by the limitations of your body in the same way my friend felt trapped by her job; but, just as she did, you have a choice. Consider your thoughts about your current lifestyle and determine if they are holding you back. Remember, what we think, we become.

ANT Therapy

Dr. Daniel Amen, a board certified psychiatrist, *New York Time's* bestselling author, and the founder of Amen Clinics in California, explained the repetitive cycle of self-talk and how to combat it with A.N.T. (automatic negative thoughts) Therapy in an American Holistic Health Association self-help article. According to Dr. Amen, "Whenever you notice these automatic negative thoughts you need to crush them or they'll ruin your relationships, your self-esteem, and your personal power." Your success depends on your ability to replace the old, negative thoughts with new, positive ones.

9 A.N.T. species include:

- **"Always" thinking: Thinking in words such as** *always, never, no one, everyone, every time*, **and** *everything*.
- **Focusing on the negative: Only seeing the bad in a situation.**
- **Fortune telling: Predicting the worst possible outcome to a situation.**
- **Mind reading: Believing that you know what another person is thinking, even though they haven't told you.**
- **Thinking with your feelings: Believing negative feelings without ever questioning them.**
- **Guilt beatings: Thinking in words such as** *should, must, ought* **or** *have to*.
- **Labeling: Attaching a negative label to yourself or to someone else.**
- **Personalization: Innocuous events are taken to have personal meaning.**
- **Blame: Blaming someone else for your own problems.**[3]

This is where we need to renew our minds. Start by listening to your inner voice, and then begin catching yourself when the old soundtrack plays. Identify any negative patterns (listed below) and create a positive, truthful, and productive inner voice. This takes time and practice. Cultivating a healthy relationship with yourself means you speak to yourself the same way you talk to your child, best friend, or someone else you love very much.

Steps to Change: Create Replacement Statements

1. Identify your negative theme and where it came from. Don't define yourself by someone else's opinion. When you choose words to describe yourself, make sure they are true of who you are now, not who you used to be. Don't blame yourself for something someone else said or did to you.
2. Replace the lies you believe about yourself with the truth of God's Word. Do you know the freedom you have available to you? Read below in "Discover Yourself in Christ" to uncover the truth about who you are.
3. Practice speaking to yourself correctly. If it helps, memorize scriptures that will strengthen you. If you wouldn't say it to your children or someone you love and respect, then you shouldn't be saying it to yourself.
4. Quickly notice and correct old thinking patterns, and pray for God to reveal when past issues resurface.

Until our thoughts change, nothing changes. It all starts with our thinking. Making a list of old, wrong thinking versus new, right thinking will help you understand the things you've allowed to repeat over and over again that aren't true. Write down how you currently talk to yourself and create a list of the common themes and new ways to begin to speak to yourself.

Discover Yourself in Christ

Do you know who you are in Christ? Maybe you have heard this question before. But do you really know what it means?

When I first became a Christian, being told I had an identity in Christ made no sense at all. I had accepted Jesus as my savior, but I didn't think He actually cared about me or wanted to know me and help me. Not really understanding his place in my life or my place in Him caused me much confusion, so (now that I have a firm grasp on this) let me share what having your identity in Him means and how that should affect your health and fitness.

First of all, if you have accepted Christ, then you have accepted a loving, compassionate, and powerful friend into your life. Jesus cares about every intimate detail of your being. He brings grace so that you may live your life to the fullest, and that includes living a healthy lifestyle.

In Christ:

- You are saved by faith from your every shortcoming. (Ephesians 2:8)
- You are made complete. (Colossians 2:10)
- You are given a fresh start. (2 Corinthians 5:17)
- You are loved. (1 John 3:3)
- You are redeemed and forgiven. (Colossians 1:14)
- You are not called to have a spirit of fear but one of love, power, and a sound mind. (2 Timothy 1:7)
- You can be confident that He who began a good work in you will be faithful to complete it. (Philippians 1:6)
- You can always know the presence of God because He will never leave you nor forsake you. (Hebrews 13:5)
- You are accepted. (Ephesians 1:6)

- You have direct access to God. (Ephesians 2:18)
- You are a temple of God because His spirit is alive in you. (1 Corinthians 6:19)
- You are a child of God. (John 1:12)
- You have the power of God working in you to accomplish the things He wants you to do. (Philippians 2:13)
- You have access to the wisdom of God when you don't know what to do. (James 1:5)

Jesus Christ has opened so many doors for us to be the confident, strong women God wants us to be. Daily struggles might come, but Jesus says we are enough in Him. In Him we can find the lasting motivation for a healthy lifestyle because of the work he has prepared for us to do. The world might tell us that looking like a supermodel will make us happy, but the only lasting joy is found in the Word of God and accepting our identity in Christ.

Don't Expect New Results From an Old Mindset.

> **And no one puts new wine into old wineskins. For the old skins would burst from the pressure, spilling the wine and ruining the skins. New wine is stored in new wineskins so that both are preserved.**
>
> **—Matthew 9:17 NLT**

I once had a client who wanted to drop fifteen pounds. It had been her desire for years, and when she came to me I knew she needed a different approach. Even with the best diet and training plan she didn't believe she could do it. She had the "how to," but she couldn't seem to shake her old way of thinking about herself and what she was capable of. One day she said, "I'm a quitter. I never finish anything." And there was the problem. As it turned out, the weight wasn't the issue. My client saw herself as a failure, and that is why she wasn't succeeding.

You can't become who you want to be if you don't change who you are.

Do you believe you can achieve your goals? I do, and God does too! But you can't become who you want to be if you don't change who you are. Your body will only do what your mind tells it to. You can change everything about your life—the way you eat, how much time you spend working out, and even your job—but if you don't change your mindset, you'll go back to the same old you.

Stop your old way of thinking and let this be the time you finish what you start. After all, you've got the best training partner. Nothing will give you more power than reflecting on and believing in who you are in Christ.

With a new mindset founded in your identity in Christ:

- See yourself as someone who can get healthy. Create a new vision of yourself and of what you're able to accomplish.
- Rise above any old level of achievement you've set. Don't limit yourself to your past personal best. Raise the bar another level. This isn't always a big event; it could be something as small as getting off the couch, going for a walk, or cooking your favorite unhealthy foods in a new and healthy way.
- Don't be afraid to present your case before the Lord. There is no reason why He would want you to be overweight, obsessed with your weight, insecure, or unhappy about yourself. Ask Him to help you find balance.

MAKE THE CHANGE

Are your thoughts robbing you of believing that you can get healthy with God? Don't you think it's time to take back your power and trade those negative thoughts for positive ones? Below are some common thought-paralyzing traps and their positive trade-ups. It's time to make the change from the world to the Word.

Trade Fear for Faith

**For God has not given us a spirit of fear and timidity,
but of power, love, and self-discipline.**
— 2 Timothy 1:7 NLT

Do you have a goal or dream that you're too afraid to go for? Perhaps someone in your past told you that you weren't smart enough or good enough and you've allowed those words to stay with you all these years, affecting not only your self-esteem but your physical ability to accomplish that task as well. Well, now it's your choice. You can believe them or start believing what God says about you.

**So do not fear, for I am with you; do not be dismayed,
for I am your God. I will strengthen you and help you;
I will uphold you with my righteous right hand.**
—Isaiah 41:10 NIV

Remember, a failure in the past doesn't make you a failure. We fail our way to success, and God strengthens us along the way.

Instead of living an unhealthy life because you're afraid to shop for healthful food or be seen at the gym, tell yourself, *God has not given me a spirit of fear and timidity, but of power, love, and self-discipline.*

Trade Guilt and Shame for Mercy and Forgiveness

Do you feel really bad about things you did in the past? Has this made you feel like you don't deserve a good life? It's a lie! I have done a number of things that I am not proud of; but, looking back on them, I know they happened so I could be shaped into who I was supposed to be. The worst thing we can do is to hide experiences in our hearts and continue to feel shame over what happened years ago. It's not about what we've done; it's about what He did once and for all.

It may not seem like your past sin is affecting your health, but it affects how you see yourself, and if it's a negative view you're clinging to, then it's holding you back. Sin makes us feel unworthy and keeps us from coming to the only one who is truly able to help.

He has removed our sins as far from us as the east is from the west.

—Psalm 103:12 NLT

If we confess our sins, he is faithful and just and will forgive us our sins and purify us from all unrighteousness.

—1 John 1:9 NIV

Don't allow the shame of past and present sin to block you from the healthy and happy life you deserve. Tell yourself every day that God will forgive your sins and purify you from all unrighteousness if you will take your guilt and shame to Him.

Trade Worry and Stress for Peace

Do you negatively meditate on things that *might* happen? Do you stress about the little things?

Our emotions can take us on a ride every day if we let them. We need to manage our stress with the Word because anxiety literally wreaks havoc on our hearts by driving up blood pressure, and it doesn't help our weight loss efforts either, as it increases a hormone called cortisol, which is responsible for belly fat. So, give your stress to God and reap the health benefits of living worry free.

Don't worry about anything; instead, pray about everything. Tell God what you need, and thank him for all he has done.

—Philippians 4:6 NLT

And the peace of God, which surpasses all understanding, will guard your hearts and minds through Christ Jesus.

—Philippians 4:7 NKJV

Whenever you're tempted to worry about your children, your husband, your job, or anything else throughout the day, pray instead. Thank God for all of these blessings, and tell Him what you need—patience, understanding, self-control.

Trade Comparison for Confidence

As women, it's easy to compare ourselves to one another. But it is wrong, and we cannot please God when we do it. Comparison goes against the Word of God because either we think we're better than someone else, which is pride, or we feel insecure, which contradicts our identity of worthiness in Christ.

God made us all in His image with different strengths and

physical attributes, and He doesn't make mistakes. Don't waste time comparing your weight to that of a celebrity you admire, your post-baby body to your sister-in-law's, your legs to those of the new woman at work, or your proportions to your best friend's. God knew exactly what He was doing when He created *you*.

> **Let everyone be sure that he is doing his very best, for then he will have the personal satisfaction of work well done and won't need to compare himself with someone else.**
>
> **—Galatians 6:4 TLB**

> **So don't lose your confidence, since it holds a great reward for you.**
>
> **—Hebrews 10:35 ISV**

The next time you want to start comparing yourself to someone else, hold on to your confidence by stating what is beautiful about another woman without putting yourself down. Notice the beauty of others around you without discounting that you have your own special qualities as well.

Trade Confusion for Clarity

In Step 1 we discussed how dieting causes division within ourselves that makes us feel defeated and so confused about what to eat or what workout to do that we end up doing nothing.

We don't just want to set our goals; we want to see them through. But when we continually break self-made promises, it erodes our confidence and breeds confusion. Therefore, believing that your honest effort will yield results, even when you haven't seen them yet, binds your mindset to peace and confidence rather than confusion and insecurity.

For God is not a God of confusion but of peace.
—1 Corinthians 14:33 ESV

All you need to say is simply "Yes" or "No"; anything beyond this comes from the evil one.
—Matthew 5:37 NIV

Trade "It's too late" for "God will do a new thing"

Have you written yourself off? If you're alive, then God isn't done with you yet. Did you know there's a purpose for your life? God has redeemed you in Christ because he has work for you to do. Being healthy and fit will prepare and equip you to accomplish that work, so find your lasting motivation for a new, healthy lifestyle in any vision or goal God has placed on your heart. This time next year you'll be so happy you chased your dreams, started your health kick, or began a new chapter of life pursuing God's purpose for you. So, get busy and see how much happier you are moving forward versus sitting around regretting you never did anything.

"For I know the plans I have for you," declares the Lord, "plans for welfare and not for evil, to give you a future and a hope."
—Jeremiah 29:11 ESV

For I am confident of this very thing, that He who began a good work in you will perfect it until the day of Christ Jesus.
—Philippians 1:6 NASB

These are just a few examples of common themes that can rob us of the life God has planned for us, but you get the idea: don't die before you're dead. The past really needs to be in the past. It's time to go forward with God and believe that, in Him, you can do anything.

I'm always overwhelmed when I read about how precious we are to God. He says that we are His masterpiece. Doesn't that amaze you? We need to remind ourselves daily of how special we are to Him. With His strength and guidance, we can believe in faith that if we do our part, then He will be with us every step of the way along this health journey.

For we are God's masterpiece. He has created us anew in Christ Jesus, so we can do the good things he planned for us long ago.

—Ephesians 2:10 NLT

GET F.I.T.

Do not be conformed to this world, but be transformed by the renewal of your mind, that by testing you may discern what is the will of God, what is good and acceptable and perfect.

—Romans 12:2 ESV

What we think about and how we speak to ourselves is important if we are going to experience a Faith Inspired Transformation. Scripture tells us that we become our thoughts, so it's important for us to filter our inner dialogue through the Word of God and practice replacement statements when negativity threatens our inner balance.

Reflection Questions:

- What thoughts are robbing you of believing you can get healthy with God?

____

____

____

- What positive trade-ups can you make to change your view from the world to the Word?

____

____

____

Practice the strategies below to renew your mind and begin making changes that will affect your health in a positive way.

Strategy #1: Understand why you do what you do. Look for the emotional component to your behavior.

- Are you eating a candy bar because you're stressed?

- Are you sabotaging your goals because you feel unworthy to reach them?
- Have you simply given up on yourself?

Strategy #2: Address what internal messages need to be changed. Arm yourself with scriptures and employ the four steps to change negative thinking.

Strategy #3: Prayerfully ask God to point out any old pain or issue that is causing a barrier between your health and happiness, and begin showering that issue in prayer.

Strategy #4: Understand that change takes time, but acknowledge that you can do anything through faith in Christ.

Strategy #5: Choose to see yourself through the Word of God. Believe that He wants to turn your health and happiness around just as much as you do.

STEP THREE | COMMIT TO THE F.I.T. POWER HOUR

Practice Spiritual, Mental, and Physical Fitness

But seek first the kingdom of God and his righteousness, and all these things will be added to you.

—Matthew 6:33 ESV

I was so frazzled trying to plan everything perfectly, running around shopping for the best gifts, and trying to make my home look like a Hallmark card that I found myself feeling really empty and miserable. I started thinking, *What is my problem? It's Christmas, and I'm stressed out and not enjoying my favorite time of year.*

A few days later I was still feeling overwhelmed and miserable, so I decided to wake up early and read my Bible. It had been weeks since I'd spent time with God, and I was disappointed in myself when I realized how easily I had fallen out of my morning routine. It was obvious that this time with God, in the Word and prayer, was the glue holding me together on a regular basis. I had been so intent on my perfect Christmas that I had been putting off my daily time with Him.

Don't we all wait to "have the time" instead of doing what we know is good for us? Well, that time will never just land in our laps. Even if we do have the time to do what's good for us, we will likely find other ways to spend it. We need to prioritize and actively make the time to do things that will bring us closer to a healthy lifestyle.

SPIRITUAL TRAINING

Create in me a clean heart, O God, and renew a right spirit within me.

—Psalm 51:10 ESV

There's something sacred about mornings. And as a mom, I've learned there's a difference when I start my day with God and when I don't. There's a structure to my life when I put Him first. I get more done, my stress level is lower, and somehow I actually have more time throughout the rest of the day. I couldn't wrap my head around the idea of getting up early in college, especially if there wasn't a test I needed to cram for. When I became a mother, however, I recognized the need for time alone in the Word first thing in the morning, before I walked out into the world. Now on the days I choose to sleep in and wake to the hectic morning rush, I'm reminded just how important a peaceful beginning to my day is.

When the inside is right, the outside will follow.

Setting aside time in the morning for spiritual training has enabled me to have the discipline to train physically in the morning as well because when the inside is right, the outside will follow.

When people think of getting fit, they tend to picture an outward transformation. The images of abs and bikini bodies are how we idealize fitness, but those results are fleeting and unfulfilling if all done in vanity. It's the inner transformation that produces lasting results.

In this sense, spiritual training as well as physical training is necessary for your overall health, but spiritual training must take the lead. Time in prayer, listening to your favorite Christian music as you work out, and remembering scriptures to help you get through whatever you're facing are all excellent ways to spiritually train yourself.

So, the question now is how will you find the time to fit God into your busy schedule?

THE F.I.T. POWER HOUR

For while bodily training is of some value, godliness is of value in every way, as it holds promise for the present life and also for the life to come.
—1 Timothy 4:8 ESV

I noticed years ago that I was a happier and healthier wife, mother, and friend on the days I spent time with God, got my workout in, and found a few reflective moments. Striving to work God, exercise, and self-reflection into my schedule every day, I began to call this time my F.I.T. Power Hour, and it has helped me find lasting health and fitness.

The F.I.T. Power Hour is a daily, one-hour commitment broken up into three twenty-minute segments that focus on spiritual, mental, and physical fitness.

The three components of the F.I.T. Power Hour are as follows:

- **F.I.T. Soul**–Time in the Word
- **F.I.T. Mind**–Time with yourself in reflection, prayer, and gratitude
- **F.I.T. Body**–Time exercising

Don't think you have to limit any of these components to twenty minutes. Your F.I.T. Power Hour can be broken up into twenty-minute increments, another combination of increments (such as five minutes in the Word, thirty-five minutes exercising, and twenty minutes in the shower praying), or combined into a single hour (in which case you might listen to the Bible on your iPod as you work out and pray at the same time).

There are days, I'll admit, that I only get in a F.I.T. Power Half Hour, and that's okay too. The goal is to make a daily commitment of spiritual, mental, and physical training. It's not about being perfect; it's about doing what you can. And something is always better than nothing.

Let's take a deeper look at the three components of the F.I.T. Power Hour.

F.I.T. Soul

Spending time in the Word is the most important thing a person can do to achieve their health and happiness goals. For many years I had it backwards. I thought if I could just make myself (and my life) perfect, I would be happy. Easy, right? Wrong! With a soul that was starved for attention, I still felt empty. And who wants to feel empty? I certainly don't anymore.

So, things are different now. I read or listen to scripture first thing every morning. I love starting my day this way because it fills me with the words of encouragement I need to keep up with a busy schedule. And since the enemy seems to make a bid for my thoughts before my feet even hit the floor, this is a habit that helps me fight fire with fire.

When it comes to F.I.T. Soul, God isn't looking for a specific amount of time each day. Ultimately, He wants to spend the whole day with us. Whatever we're doing, He wants to come along and help direct, guide, and enable us. However, sometimes we are the ones who need to get used to the idea of spending time with Him. Therefore, the twenty minutes or so we devote to God as a part of our F.I.T. Power Hour prepares our hearts to allow Him in and reminds us to carry Him with us wherever we go and to turn to Him with our every problem.

Struggling with food all my life, I never realized how impactful time spent with God was until I asked Him to help me overcome my overeating and emotional eating. He helped me hit the pause button and find a passion to make the right choices. I started asking myself questions such as, *Am I really hungry? How will I feel after eating this?* and *What is a healthy alternative I could try?* Asking such questions helped me think about how much I was eating and inspired me to learn how to cook my favorite meals in a healthy way.

Finding time to read the Bible (our manual for life) may seem like a challenge, but it's easily accomplished in a number of ways.

F.I.T. Soul Tips:

- **Begin the day reading the Bible with your morning coffee or tea.**
- **Get a verse-of-the-day app on your phone.**
- **Watch inspirational Christian video lessons from teachers such as Joyce Meyer and T.D. Jakes.**
- **Put Christian music, books, and the Bible on your iPod or iPad and read or listen:**
- **In the school pick up line;**
- **Waiting for appointments;**
- **On your lunch break; and**
- **During your daily commute.**
- **End your day reflecting on scripture.**

I believe God would prefer that we remember one verse than spend an hour reading and not remember anything. Our journey with God is personal and beautiful. He desires relationship without any guilt on our end, so if you have only five minutes, then that's good enough for God. In fact, He can do more in five minutes than you could ever imagine.

F.I.T. Mind

Our mind is where we win or lose every day because that is where all of the little choices we make add up to determine the course of our lives. Joyce Meyer's book *Battlefield of the Mind* sums it up in just a title because our mind really can be like a battlefield with the world waging war against the Word of God to determine our thoughts.

Picture a dial with the Word on one side and the world on the other. Where would you be positioned on this dial? Our daily F.I.T. Mind goal is to move that dial more toward the Word and away from the world. Today it is commonplace for us to make idols out of promotions, lifestyles, and people. From careers to weight loss, we allow that far-reaching goal to drive and define us. But whatever consumes our thoughts is taking up space in that special place where only God should reside.

When I was working to get published as a model, getting on a magazine cover was my idol. I'm embarrassed to admit that I was obsessed with it and it took the number one position in my mind—way before God. How I felt about myself was dictated by the magazine's yes or no, and I saw myself as a success or failure based on their opinion. But the only opinion that ever really matters is our Lord's. That's why we've got to turn that dial in the right direction!

What's defining you right now? If you take that imposed view off of yourself and see through God's eyes, you'll immediately feel liberated from "what they think." The world is always trying to tell us how we should feel about ourselves, which (as we learned in Step 2) makes spending time in the Word invaluable. The Word teaches us where we get our value from, and it isn't in our weight, how few calories we're able to consume in a day, or any other single determining factor; it's in our Savior.

Start checking in with yourself on a daily basis. There is a constant battle to keep us from the peace and joy that only God can give. And, when we aren't dealing with our emotions, we may end up eating for comfort and engaging in self-destructive behaviors that actually sabotage our goals and our health. Daily "check-ins" can prevent these behaviors from spinning out of control.

Journaling your thoughts and feelings and spending time in reflection and gratitude, are effective ways you may check in with yourself. Clearly understanding why you're feeling what you're feeling goes a long way in moving that dial toward the Word and away from the world, thus producing a happy, healthy, and blessed life.

F.I.T. Mind Tips:

- **Commit to five minutes of journaling first thing in the morning, during your coffee break, or at night before bed.**
- **Spend time getting to know yourself and your triggers.**
- **Pray/read scriptures that support you in whatever you're going through.**
- **If the Bible intimidates you, simply Google what the Bible says about whatever you're going through, and you'll be amazed at the life-changing help you'll find.**
- **Use the replacement strategies in Step 2 to undo any thoughts that are not from God. Practice speaking to yourself the way you would to someone you greatly love and respect, and undo any health-stealing negativity you've been putting up with.**

Your F.I.T. Mind time can be accomplished any time of day. I like to tuck myself in at night with a bit of journaling. Checking in with myself

Dream big, plan, reflect, pray, and know in faith that God is working in your life.

clears my mind and prepares me for a restful night of sleep. I recommend handwriting in a journal because there is a personal connection that forms between you and your little book. It holds your dreams and prayers, and, in time, you will be able to look back at your entries and see just how far you've come.

F.I.T. Body

Training

As a working mom, there isn't any extra time during the day, so I have to make time early in the morning for exercise. Sometimes it seems impossible to tear myself from my comfortable, warm bed, so I keep my headphones and iPod on my nightstand in order to plug in and listen to the Bible or Christian music as soon as my alarm goes off at 5 a.m. As I make my morning tea and get ready to work out, I'm already in my own little world, praising God and feeling empowered by His Spirit. I've actually come to enjoy this routine and look forward to it each day.

Because time is a precious commodity, combining my workouts with the Word is my solution to a time-crunched schedule (and it reminds me to have faith as I pursue lasting fitness). I can get in a great workout while listening to a whole chapter or more of the Bible. On days when I need the energy music brings, I begin and cool down in the Word, and in between I've got some great Christian music—Mandisa, Jeremy Camp, Casting Crowns, Vaughaligan Walwyn, Lecrae, Third Day, and Toby Mac—to pump up my workouts, which might include fitness DVDs, running either outside or on my treadmill, lifting weights, and/or attending group fitness classes.

Working out takes serious commitment, whether we choose to do it first thing in the morning, during our lunch breaks, intermittently throughout the day, right after work, or after everyone else has gone to bed. In Step 4 we will look into the different ways in which we strengthen our bodies, but first we need to get in the habit of fitting some sort of physical activity into our schedules.

Here are a few ways in which you might begin to set a standard of daily physical exercise for yourself:

- Get up and get moving! Begin your day with a walk, jog, run, or use any DVDs (including the F.I.T. DVD series) or other equipment you have.
- Check out the free videos on YouTube for well-known programs such as P90X and many others. You can play them right from your computer and, in most cases, they can be done in small spaces.
- Work out on your lunch break.
- Schedule time to go to the gym before or after work.
- Take a new class at a local gym, YMCA, or community center and invite a friend. Trying something new can help you connect with your inner-athlete.
- Get the family moving. Bike rides, walks after dinner, and playing in the backyard are ways to increase activity that lead to a healthier lifestyle.
- Check event boards in your community's gathering places or use an Internet search engine to find local Saturday-morning hiking, biking, or jogging groups.
- Sign up your family to take classes at the local YMCA or fitness center. There are many ways to get moving, but do what you love and you'll be more likely to stick with it.

There are many perks to making exercise a part of daily life. Perhaps you've heard about the endorphin release (also referred to as a runner's high) that occurs at the end of a workout. These post-exercise hormones, often called "happy hormones" make your energy levels seem limitless, suppress your appetite, alleviate stress, and may be the best pick-me-up you'll find. Endorphins are a great reminder that this journey is supposed to be fun and make you feel great. Don't trick yourself into thinking exercise is supposed to be terrible.

FIND THE TIME

Making the best use of your time because the times are evil.

—Ephesians 5:16 ISV

As you begin to implement the F.I.T. Power Hour into your daily life, you may still find yourself crunched for time. However, I challenge you to reevaluate how you spend your time and to look for ways to build an hour back into your day. Below are ten examples of possible ways to find extra time in your schedule.

1. Go to bed earlier and wake up earlier. Set your iPod and shoes next to your bed if you are trying to work out in the morning.
2. Go on an Internet diet. Start managing the amount of time you spend on social media, playing games, and checking email. If you're not reading your Bible, spending time in prayer, or exercising because you're posting on Facebook, Twitter, Pinterest, and/or Instagram instead, you're out of balance.
3. Plan meals and cook in bulk. This is a great time-saver. On Sundays I cook while I'm doing laundry and relaxing with my family. This builds hours back into my week. Also, try packing food the night before to alleviate the morning rush. Having

healthy snacks and lunch from home saves time, money, and calories.

4. Clearly know your priorities for each day and discipline yourself to focus on getting these things done.
5. Get organized. Choose a method for organization—apps, dry erase boards, and good old-fashioned planners. Take care of yourself by planning your day in advance and allowing for a little wiggle room in your otherwise hectic schedule.
6. Be present and fight distractions. Saving time isn't necessarily about doing something faster; it's about getting it done right in the least amount of time. Give the task at hand 100 percent of your attention and then move on.
7. Listen on the go. Put your Bible and books on your iPod and listen to them while you're driving, waiting at appointments or in the school pick-up line, or working out. This is a great way to maximize gap time in your schedule and to complete your F.I.T. Power Hour.
8. Spend less time in the mirror with a quick, go-to routine. Find a makeup artist at the mall (one who gets your look) and a hair stylist to learn tips and tricks that will shave time off your morning routine. For example, a side braid or messy bun with a braided wrap make you look effortlessly put together. Learning to make yourself look your best makes you feel great, and it doesn't need to take hours.
9. Find Balance in Relationships. Not to sound harsh, but this is your life, and you're called to great things, so you can't afford to be held back with negativity or draining relationships. Spending hours on the phone and having the same-old conversations isn't helping anyone. I urge you to prayerfully consider whether or not your relationships are helping you lead your happiest and healthiest life.
10. Take the perfection pressure off. Workouts don't have to be hours long. The only bad workout is the one you didn't do. Do what you can with the time you have. So many people email me

and say they don't have time to work out because they don't have hours of free time, but no one does. Believe it or not, you can give yourself the workout of a lifetime in twenty minutes.

Prioritize

Do you ever feel as though you are chasing a to-do list? Until you have clearly defined priorities, life is going to feel like you're trapped on a hamster wheel. I felt this way during my first corporate job until I attended a Stephen Covey seminar. His organizational wisdom changed my life, and his Rocks and Sand analogy is a great reminder to me that I can always find time if I prioritize.

Rocks and Sand

Dr. Stephen Covey's rocks and sand analogy tells of an expert who stood in front of a group of business students one day and announced it was time for a quiz. He pulled out a one-gallon, wide-mouthed mason jar and set it on a table in front of him. Next he produced about a dozen fist-sized rocks and carefully placed them, one at a time, into the jar.

When the jar was filled to the top and no more rocks would fit inside, he asked, "Is this jar full?"

Everyone in the class said, "Yes."

"Really?" He asked.

Reaching under the table, he pulled out a bucket of gravel, dumped it in, and shook the jar, causing pieces of gravel to work themselves down into the spaces between the big rocks.

Then he smiled and asked the group once more, "Is the jar full?"

By this time the class was on to him.

"Probably not," one of them answered.

"Good!" he replied.

Reaching under the table, the expert brought out a bucket of sand. He started dumping the sand in and it went into all the spaces left between the rocks and the gravel. Once more he asked the question, "Is this jar full?"

"No!" the class shouted.

Once again he said, "Good!"

Then he grabbed a pitcher of water and began to pour it in until the jar was filled to the brim. Then he looked up at the class and asked, "What is the point of this illustration?"

One eager beaver raised his hand and said, "The point is that no matter how full your schedule is, if you try really hard, you can always fit some more things into it!"

"No," he replied, "that's not the point. This illustration teaches us that if you don't put the big rocks in first, you'll never get them in at all."[4]

Is getting healthy one of the big rocks in your life? What about making time for God? Remember to put these big rocks in first or you'll never get them in at all. Each day should be dedicated and planned around your big rocks.

Building your F.I.T. Power Hour into your day will set you on the course for faith-inspired living and provide the daily check-in to steer you back on track when need be. Believing we can achieve our goals with God is important in our Faith Inspired Transformation, but we need to remember that our motivation for those specific goals must be lasting. Asking God for His help to get on the cover of *Sports Illustrated* Swimsuit Edition is probably not the desire He is eager to give us because, ultimately, our greatest desire should be to love God and be more like Him. While a healthy weight and healthy body might go hand in hand with that, we need to remember to prioritize our lives. God should be the biggest rock in our F.I.T. jar, and we must change on the inside before we worry about changing the outside.

F.I.T. POWER HOUR

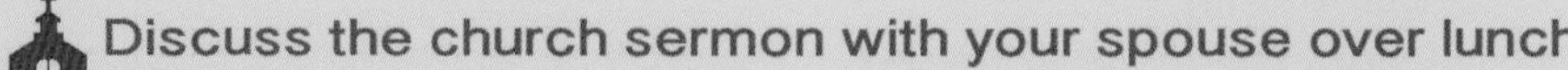

SUNDAY	Discuss the church sermon with your spouse over lunch. Take a walk after dinner. Journal before bed about anything that has been troubling you. Google what the Bible says about those things.
MONDAY	Wake up early and exercise to a fitness DVD. Listen to the Bible in the car on the way to work. Write in your journal during lunch about your goals for the week.
TUESDAY	Go for a thirty-minute jog or use cardio equipment at home while listening to the Bible or Christian music on your iPod. Take a bath and write in your journal before bed about a dream God put in your heart and three steps you can take to make it happen.
WEDNESDAY	Wake up early and read the Bible. Journal during lunch about any negative thoughts. Take a fun class after work with friends, such as barre, kickboxing, Crossfit, or Zumba.
THURSDAY	Meet a friend at the gym before work and train together. Attend a women's Bible study. Journal about your F.I.T. journey in the pick-up line at your child's school and ask God to help you get healthy for good.
FRIDAY	Do an at-home DVD workout. Write five things you're grateful for in your journal. Listen to the Bible or Christian music while driving.
SATURDAY	Wake up early to read the Bible and journal your thoughts about how what you read applies to your life. Go for a bike ride with your family.

GET F.I.T.

The F.I.T. Power Hour is a one-hour commitment to spend time getting spiritually, mentally, and physically fit. By spending time in the Word, time checking in with ourselves, and time in exercise, we are better able to see ourselves through the eyes of God as we pursue health as a Godly lifestyle. When we prioritize our time and put our spiritual, mental, and physical health first, we have the spirit of self-control to rely on rather than our weak willpower.

Reflection Questions:

- What are the "big rocks" that you are putting first in your life right now? Are they honoring to God?

  ____

  ____

  ____

- How could you prioritize your day to include an hour of spiritual, mental, and physical training? (Remember, you can combine these into one or break them up into time increments that work for you.)

  ____

  ____

  ____

Your F.I.T. Power Hour can easily become a part of your day. Try the plan on page 50 and modify it as necessary to work with your weekly schedule.

Building your F.I.T. Power Hour into your day will set you on the course for faith-inspired living and provide the daily check-in to steer you back on track when need be.

STEP FOUR | DRESS YOURSELF WITH STRENGTH

Put on "Godfidence"

She dresses herself with strength and makes her arms strong.

—Proverbs 31:17 ESV

Now that we've discovered how to make daily exercise a part of our lives with the F.I.T. Power Hour, let's explore the different ways in which we might build our physical and spiritual strength during this time. The Proverbs 31 woman is a great example of how and why we should pursue strength and fitness in our daily lives.

- She's good and faithful to her husband. (Proverbs 31:12)
- She works eagerly and vigorously. (Proverbs 31:13)
- She chooses only the choicest foods. (Proverbs 31:14)
- She gets up while it's still dark and prepares food for her family. (Proverbs 31:15)
- She is not hasty in her decisions. (Proverbs 31:16)
- Her body is strong. (Proverbs 31:17)
- She opens her arms to the poor and helps the needy. (Proverbs 31:20)
- She clothes herself with dignity. (Proverbs 31:25)
- She speaks with wisdom. (Proverbs 31:26)
- She is not lazy. (Proverbs 31:27)
- Her children and husband call her blessed. (Proverbs 31: 28)

My favorite characteristic of the Proverbs 31 woman is her strength: "She Dresses herself with strength and makes her arms strong." To dress means to clothe one's self or to put on a covering of some sort. Putting on our identity in Christ, therefore, is how we dress ourselves with internal strength—affecting the mind and spirit.

Getting Strong with Godfidence

My help comes from the Lord, the Maker of heaven and earth.

—Psalm 121:2 NIV

Our internal strength that comes from God helps us to meet each day boldly. When we put on our identity in Christ (I call it "Godfidence") we know who we are and whose we are. Jesus rose early. He walked everywhere. He prayed alone. Aiming to be like Him and learning to walk in His ways bring us to the purpose of the Faith Inspired Transformation and the F.I.T. Power Hour.

Finally, be strong in the Lord and in the strength of His might. Put on the whole armor of God, that you may be able to stand against the schemes of the devil.

—Ephesians 6:10-11 ESV

As our minds and spirits are strengthened to believe and act on the truth of who we are in Christ, we must also strengthen our bodies to fulfill the purposes God has given each of us, whether it is mission work in a foreign country; working with the disadvantaged in our local communities; helping our churches with childcare, teen events, or maintenance; or serving our families by working in the yard, cleaning the house, buying and preparing food, and chasing our children around every day.

FOUNDATION FOR FITNESS

Along with making us able-bodied and in tune with the spirit to fulfill a myriad of purposes God gives us, the body portion of our F.I.T. Power Hour is strengthening our hearts and increasing our physical strength for life in general. According to the Centers for Disease Control and Prevention, "People who are physically active for about 7 hours a week have a 40 percent lower risk of dying early than those who are active for less than 30 minutes a week."[5] Think about that—just seven hours of your week could be the difference between meeting your grandchildren or not.

With the different reasons for why we should seek fitness in mind, let's explore the different ways in which we may strengthen our bodies through cardiovascular exercise and strength training.

Why We Need Cardio

Cardiovascular (or cardio) exercise can be either aerobic or anaerobic. Aerobic exercise requires oxygen and increases the strength and endurance of the heart by elevating our heart rates and breathing for sustained periods of time. Aerobic activities such as running, jogging, dancing, cycling, swimming, and hiking (and many more) can be performed every day.

Anaerobic exercise, on the other hand, literally means "without oxygen." Anaerobic activity is going all out for short intervals of time so your heart rate goes to a near max and then drops back down to an aerobic level. This type of training increases power and speed. Anaerobic exercises (plyometrics, sprinting, high-intensity weightlifting, etc.) build strength and should be performed in accordance with your fitness level, working your way up to a minimum of twice a week.

Combining Strength Training and Cardio

Many of our daily activities require a strong body—taking the stairs, bending over, squatting down, and lifting heavier objects. Strength training (also called resistance training) is a type of exercise that increases anaerobic endurance, muscle size, bone density, fat loss, and metabolism. Because it strengthens bones and muscles, strength training may also prevent injury when done properly. Weights, body weight, resistance bands, therabands, kettlebells, TRX suspension trainers, exercise balls, medicine balls, and even sleds are equipment that may be used in strength training.

Cardio and strength training can be performed separately or together. One method in which they may be done together is in circuit training, which combines both aerobic and anaerobic exercises with resistance training. Circuits are a series of exercises performed one after the other (in a circuit) with minimal rest in-between. Circuit training is a great answer to a limited amount of time when you are working out at home or traveling.

For beginners combining strength training and cardio, cardio in an aerobic range can be performed every day of the week. The goal is to get your heart rate up for at least twenty minutes a day. This can be combined with introductory strength training exercises: push-ups, squats, and lunges. A great place to begin is to hire a trainer to teach proper form and demonstrate how different machines should be used.

If you are on a time-crunched schedule, try the F.I.T. DVD circuit series. This DVD series comes with beginner, intermediate, and advanced workouts that combine cardio with functional strength training (your body weight or five pound dumbbells) to get the most out of your workout. Each workout also includes a F.I.T. mind challenge, an inspiring message, and a scripture to spiritually strengthen you.

Run Your Race

> **So I run with purpose in every step. I am not just shadowboxing. I discipline my body like an athlete, training it to do what it should. Otherwise, I fear that after preaching to others I myself might be disqualified.**
> **—1 Corinthians 9:26-27 NLT**

Regardless of where you are on the spectrum of fitness, remember to run *your* race. We all start somewhere, and the victors are the ones who don't give up.

Have you ever trained for a long-distance race? These types of sporting events are just as much about mental toughness as they are about physical ability. Think about it. When a marathon runner is nearing mile twenty-five, and their legs begin to cramp so badly that they wince with pain at every step, do you think they're going to just give in and say, "Well, I'm done. I'll try again tomorrow." Of course not! Most likely that runner has been training for months—waking up early every morning to run before work and mixing grueling speed workouts with extremely long runs that might have pushed them to the brink of boredom. At mile twenty-five it doesn't matter how loudly their flesh is screaming for them to quit because that runner is going to give it everything to make the final mile.

Now, I'm not saying everyone should work out to the point of injury or distaste in a particular activity. I'm saying that, if you're an athlete, you can't live by what your body wants. You must follow specific guidelines, not the changing desires of your body, and you let your well-informed mind dictate what your body does or does not do—you exercise when you'd rather rest; you eat healthy, balanced food when you would rather eat fast food; you sleep when you would rather stay up late; and you get up early to train when you would rather stay in bed.

Learn from the example of the athlete and bring your body under your control. Clothe yourself with strength and make your arms (and legs) strong for the race set before you.

Challenge Yourself

Don't you realize that in a race everyone runs, but only one person gets the prize? So run to win!

—1 Corinthians 9:24 NLT

So, how hard do you need to work out?

When it comes to determining how hard you need to push yourself, it's important that you first know how hard your heart is already working compared to how hard it should be working. This will give you an idea of your current fitness level.

To determine what your resting heart rate is:

- **find your pulse on the inside of your wrist, the side that your thumb is on;**
- **use the tips of your pointer and middle fingers and gently press on the blood vessels of your wrist;**
- **hold for ten seconds, counting the number of pulsations, and multiply that number by six to find your beats per minute.[6]**

There are also many heart rate monitor watches you can wear while you exercise. Choose which method works best for you. Periodically checking the number is inspiring and can be used as motivation to push yourself. The more you work out, the lower your resting heart rate will be. This is a sign that your heart is working more efficiently.

If you're new to exercise, check with your doctor to make sure you're in good health before beginning a new workout regimen. Once you've been cleared, or if you're in great health, safely challenge yourself in your workouts by aiming for a heart rate zone (use charts below) that corresponds to your fitness goals and maintaining that heart rate at the proper intensity level (between 50 to 85 percent of your maximum heart rate) for at least 20 minutes.

THE RIGHT INTENSITY

Find Your Target Zone

AGE	65-75% of Max Heart Rate Light to Moderate	75-85% of Max Heart Rate Moderate to Heavy
20	130 - 150	150 - 170
25	127 - 146	146 - 166
30	123 - 142	142 - 161
35	120 - 138	138 - 157
40	117 - 135	135 - 153
45	114 - 131	131 - 149
50	110 - 127	127 - 144
55	107 - 124	124 - 140
60	104 - 120	120 - 136
65	101 - 116	116 - 132
70	97 - 112	112 - 127

You need to challenge yourself to build strength. Never push yourself beyond a healthy boundary, but don't slack either. Listen to your body and give your workout your best effort. It will be difficult, maybe even painful, but if it doesn't challenge you, it doesn't change you.

If it doesn't challenge you, it doesn't change you.

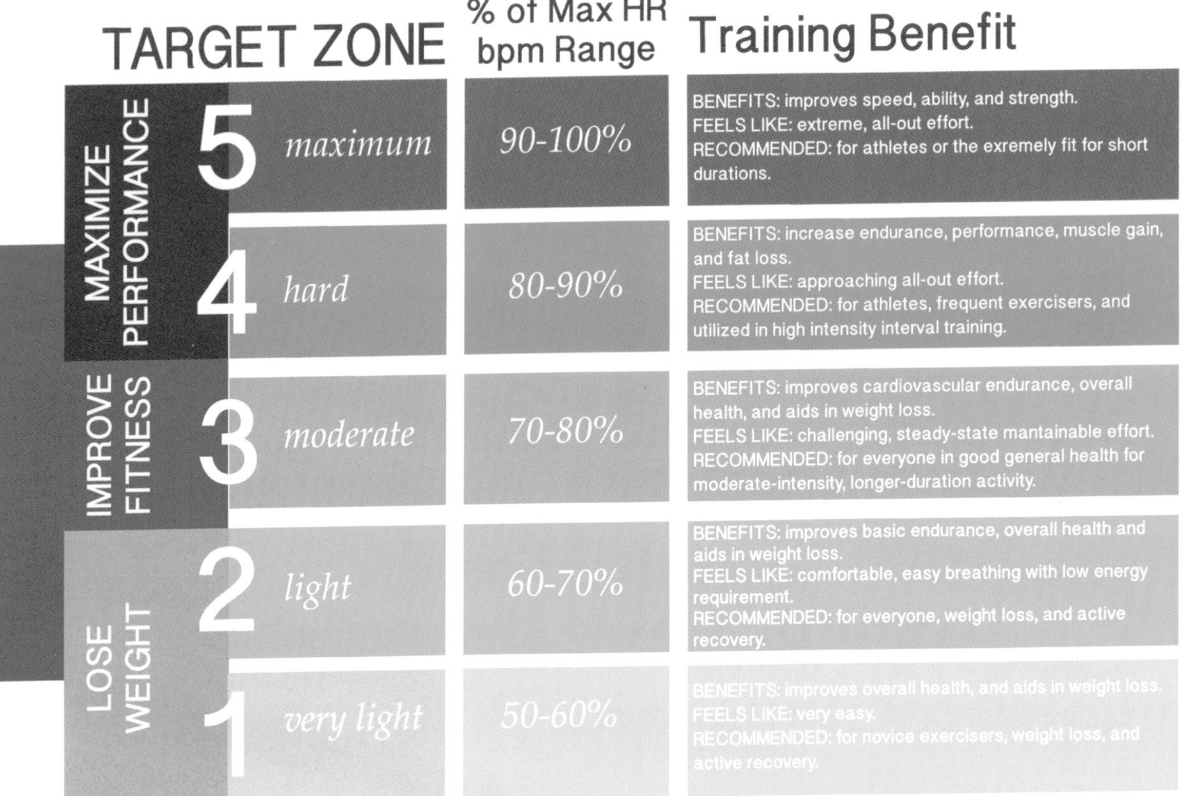

	TARGET ZONE		% of Max HR bpm Range	Training Benefit
MAXIMIZE PERFORMANCE	5	*maximum*	*90-100%*	BENEFITS: improves speed, ability, and strength. FEELS LIKE: extreme, all-out effort. RECOMMENDED: for athletes or the exremely fit for short durations.
	4	*hard*	*80-90%*	BENEFITS: increase endurance, performance, muscle gain, and fat loss. FEELS LIKE: approaching all-out effort. RECOMMENDED: for athletes, frequent exercisers, and utilized in high intensity interval training.
IMPROVE FITNESS	3	*moderate*	*70-80%*	BENEFITS: improves cardiovascular endurance, overall health, and aids in weight loss. FEELS LIKE: challenging, steady-state mantainable effort. RECOMMENDED: for everyone in good general health for moderate-intensity, longer-duration activity.
LOSE WEIGHT	2	*light*	*60-70%*	BENEFITS: improves basic endurance, overall health and aids in weight loss. FEELS LIKE: comfortable, easy breathing with low energy requirement. RECOMMENDED: for everyone, weight loss, and active recovery.
	1	*very light*	*50-60%*	BENEFITS: improves overall health, and aids in weight loss. FEELS LIKE: very easy. RECOMMENDED: for novice exercisers, weight loss, and active recovery.

Take the Work Out of Workout

Although a well-balanced exercise plan includes cardio and strength training, the best workout you can give yourself is something you enjoy doing. For a moment, contemplate something you've always wanted to do. It could be hiking a mountain, running a marathon, taking a dance class, or even tackling a lofty goal like a fitness competition. The benefits of exercise are endless, but you need to find what you love doing. Exercise should be stress relieving and energy producing. If you dread it, think about how to change it.

I recently hit a wall with my training. I began to loathe going to the gym and decided to try group fitness classes. These classes renewed my excitement and made me look forward to working out again. The social aspect of making new friends and experiencing fitness together was something that made me want to keep going back.

If you're stuck in an exercise rut, try something new that will renew your enthusiasm for fitness.

Is Your "But" Too Big?

I want to work out, *but* I don't have enough time.
I wish I could work out, *but* I don't have the money.
I worked out for a month, *but* I didn't notice any changes.

Excuse-proofing your workout means you focus on finding a solution and take the "but" out of your exercise vocabulary. When it comes to working out, the word *but* is usually followed by an excuse or rationalization. The list of why we can't fit it into our day can be exhaustive. I've heard every excuse in the world, and I have to admit I've made them myself. My favorites include: "As soon as I drop a few pounds, I'll get back to the gym," and, of course, "I'm too busy!"

Here are examples, once more, of how easy it is to crush an excuse to not work out:

- Get up just twenty-five minutes earlier and go for a walk or jog, pop in an exercise DVD, or do cardio on your home equipment (treadmill, stationary bike, elliptical).
- Take a group class or even a walk on your lunch break.
- Pick two days a week and meet your friends at barre, yoga, or a boot camp.
- Take a walk or bike ride after dinner.
- Watch your favorite TV show while you do sit-ups and push-ups.
- Play tag, dodgeball, hopscotch, or create an obstacle course outside with your kids.

- Go for family bike rides, hikes, or swims on the weekends.
- Knock out household chores, clean out the garage, garden, or wash the car.

Don't let your "but" get too big!

If you're just starting out on your fitness journey, adding exercise to your day might require an adjustment or two, but there are simple, relatively painless ways to fit it in. As we touched on in Step 3, instead of one session of twenty minutes, try breaking your workout into two sessions of ten minutes or four sessions of five minutes. Dividing exercise across the day is a very doable approach when spare time is in short supply.

Don't skip your workout because you're looking for the perfect time. Do what you can when you can. Make a way, not an excuse. Don't let your "but" get too big!

When the Going Gets Tough

And let us not grow weary of doing good, for in due season we will reap, if we do not give up.

—Galatians 6:9 ESV

Transforming my unhealthy, overweight body was not easy, so I fully understand the frustration and the temptation to give up. But I also know what it feels like to be on the other side of the battle, and my prayer is that you will know such freedom as well.

God desires health for you, so don't quit on yourself and don't stop believing that he will bless your efforts. Look at the following benefits of exercise. With a list like this, how could you deny that God doesn't desire a F.I.T. body for you?

TOP 10 BENEFITS OF EXERCISE

1. Exercise lengthens your life span and prevents many diseases, such as heart disease, high blood pressure, abnormal blood lipid (cholesterol and triglyceride) profile, type 2 diabetes, metabolic syndrome, and colon and breast cancers.
2. Exercise makes you strong and improves your fitness level.
3. Exercise raises your metabolism and helps you lose weight.
4. Exercise reduces stress, anxiety, and depression.
5. Exercise is beneficial for brain health.
6. Exercise aids in healthy digestion.
7. Exercise increases bone density.
8. Exercise provides fresh oxygenated blood throughout your body, which makes you age gracefully and keeps you agile.
9. Exercise improves sleep quality.
10. Exercise enhances your overall quality of life by boosting your mood and filling you with energy.

GET F.I.T.

But they who wait for the Lord shall renew their strength; they shall mount up with wings like eagles; they shall run and not be weary; they shall walk and not faint.

—Isaiah 40:31 ESV

Is your "but" too big? God has made us all unique and given us all a passion for some form of exercise (even if it changes from time to time). In Step 4 we learned the difference between aerobic and anaerobic exercise and the benefits of each. We also learned about finding our target heart rate zones to challenge ourselves during our workouts. Regardless of where we are with our physical fitness, the Proverbs 31 woman teaches us that we need to be sure to clothe ourselves with our identity in Christ as we make our bodies strong.

Reflection Questions:

- What excuses are holding you back from getting fit?

  ____

  ____

  ____

- What are some exercises you would enjoy doing or that you could creatively fit into your schedule in order to eliminate your excuses?

  ____

  ____

  ____

Use the strategies on the next page to get started on and stick with a workout program you enjoy.

GET F.I.T.

Strategy #1: Schedule active breaks throughout your workday. Working out isn't limited to the gym. After you've been working for a few hours at home or the office, get up, walk around, do some lunges, jumping jacks, sit ups—do anything fun to get your heart rate up. If you're a stay-at-home mom, play some great Christian music and clean your house. Make faith and fitness your way of life.

Strategy #2: Treat your workout like an appointment. We rarely miss work or doctor's appointments, but taking care of ourselves through exercise gets swept under the rug so often. Working out first thing in the morning is a great way to ensure it happens because there are too many reasons why it won't get done at the end of the day. Whatever days and times you choose, commit to them.

Strategy #3: Be daring. Take the dance or boxing class you've always been afraid of. Get off your designated cardio machine and try something new. The same-old workout makes the same-old body. Challenge yourself with new workouts that target different muscle groups than you're used to. Don't be intimidated to try something different. We all feel uncomfortable and out of place those first few times, but you've got Godfidence!

Strategy #4: Think progress, not perfection. Celebrate your successes. There is no such thing as perfection, so think progress, not perfection. If you used to be able to do five push-ups and now you can do ten, it's time to pat yourself on the back. Don't throw in the towel if you missed a day. I love the quote "Never quit on a bad day" because we all have bad days now and then, and we shouldn't let them define us.

Strategy #5: Excuse-proof your workout. Have a plan for when your day goes sideways because this is life and it will happen. If you like to work out at the gym, have a go-to home workout. Utilize online videos, DVDs, and fitness apps to stay on track when your day doesn't go as planned.

God desires health for you, so don't quit on yourself and don't stop believing that he will bless your efforts.

STEP FIVE | SET F.A.I.T.H. GOALS

Plan for Success

When Jesus saw him lying there and learned that he had been in this condition for a long time, he asked him, "Do you want to get well?"... Then Jesus said to him, "Get up! Pick up your mat and walk." At once the man was cured; he picked up his mat and walked.

John 5:6, 8–9 NIV

This man had been lying next to a healing pool for thirty-eight years. Yet, even with the answer to his ailment so close to him, he never got in the water. Perhaps he couldn't walk, but surely he could have moved a little at a time or asked someone for help.

When Jesus asked the man if he wanted to get well, I think we normally tend to believe that Jesus already knew his answer and was just teasing him before bringing the healing, but think about it: Jesus asked him if he wanted to get well, He saw the man's condition and let him know that he had to make the choice.

Do you want to get well? Picture your life. Think of the issues you have dealt with that kept you on the sidelines and denied you health and happiness—depression, anxiety, fear, self-loathing. How long did you stay there? Are you still there? Just like the lame man by the healing pool, you have the option to get well. The only catch is that you too must get up and move. Jesus told him, "Get Up!" Is getting up all that's holding you back?

Setting F.A.I.T.H. goals is the way we can get up and get moving toward health and happiness. However, we often make excuses. I know I do at times. My go-to excuse is that I don't have enough time. In fact, with a packed work schedule and the responsibility of taking care of our home and our daughter, I have to fight the excuse of "I don't have enough time" quite often.

I think we all like to believe that it's easier for other people to pursue health and fitness goals, but I know this is not the case because we all get the same twenty-four hours in a day and we've all dealt with difficult issues. God has really helped me grow up and "get up" when I hear myself saying I don't have enough time because what I'm really saying is that I'm choosing to make an excuse rather than find a way.

Just as I'm not the only one with a busy schedule, I know I'm not the only one who needs to find a way either. We all need to turn our words into actions. We have spent the past few steps ditching diets, changing our mindsets, and building time into our day for spiritual, mental, and physical fitness. Now that we have established a foundation, we can begin to put our knowledge into practice by setting F.A.I.T.H. goals.

SET F.A.I.T.H. GOALS

A goal without a plan is just a wish.
— Antoine de Saint-Exupery

As I mentioned before, God is more than willing to help us achieve a Faith Inspired Transformation, but we still need to do some of the work ourselves. For this reason, setting personal goals is vital to our success. Have you ever put your health goals in writing? I don't mean writing your ideal weight on a piece of paper that taunts you until it is conveniently lost. No, I'm talking about sitting down with a pen and paper and making a tangible, feasible list of health and fitness goals.

Dr. Gail Matthews, a psychology professor at Dominican University in California, found that people are 42% more likely to achieve their goals if they're written down. However, it's hard to achieve a goal with no clear direction other than a number. Therefore, as a way to keep your motivations in check and set a clear course for your F.I.T. success, I've created the F.A.I.T.H. acronym.

F - Faith-Filled and Specific
A - Accountable
I - Inspiring
T - Time-Based and Measurable
H - Healthy

Faith-filled and Specific

Seek God first and pray for wisdom to make God-led goals. We never want to get ahead of God, but we need to act. Nothing will happen by just sitting around. We take a step in faith, stay in prayer, and allow Him to direct our paths. Picture a marathon runner nearing the end of the race. They don't accidently trip across the finish line, and neither will we. We won't stumble upon success; we have to achieve it.

Our success is brought about through the daily decisions we make, and good decisions are easier to make when they are set in faith and clearly defined. Ask God for wisdom, and then answer these specific questions:

- What is your goal? (Example: You could hope to go down a dress size, lower your cholesterol, or gain muscle.)
- How will you accomplish it? (Example: You could either work out alone or with a friend or a trainer. You could work out in a gym or at home.)
- What are the reasons, purposes, and benefits of achieving your goal? (Example: Do you want to live a long life for your children;

would you like to run a marathon; are you trying to fit back into your favorite jeans; or are you just sick of feeling bad about yourself?)

Accountable

Accountability is what gets you to the finish line. It's that daily focus that feeds your motivation. Accountability is the date on the calendar that you're training for, it's found in a trusted person you've agreed to work out with or a trainer you meet with and who takes your measurements every Wednesday. When you have to answer to something or someone, you excuse-proof your plan and get things done.

What are some ways to incorporate accountability in your health goals?

- Find an accountability partner and consider tracking your measurements together. This could mean weighing yourselves each week, recording your waist, hip, and thigh measurements, or trying on pieces of clothing for one another that you have been unable to fit into for a while.
- Sign up for a 5K, 10K, or perhaps a half marathon with a group or a friend and ask those people to hold you accountable to your training.
- Organize your co-workers or church group to get healthy by taking classes or going to the gym together.
- Create a blog and begin journaling your way to success by bringing people with you on your journey. Find encouragement from them and be an encouragement to them.

Inspiring

Inspiration can motivate us even through the toughest days, so keep inspiration in front of you. Make an inspiration board and fill it with things that will encourage you to press on toward achieving your goals—verses, quotes, a list of your health goals, pictures of your kids, and more. Having had my daughter later in life inspires me to eat right and exercise. My goal is to be the healthiest I can be because I want to be here for her as long as possible.

- What inspires you to get healthy? (Example: Your children, your spouse, or a lifelong dream that requires a certain level of physical ability might inspire you toward a healthy lifestyle.)
- What physical activity did you enjoy or dream of doing as a child? It's not too late to have fun again. Fitness isn't limited to the weight room and stationary equipment. (Example: I learned gymnastics in my 30s because it is something I always wanted to do. You could learn karate, kickboxing, tennis, or even join a soccer or basketball team.)
- Inspire health around you and give back. Inspiration is contagious. Invite a friend who needs cheering up or someone who needs help getting fit to join you. Nothing is more inspiring than motivating someone else.
- Load your iPod with inspirational music, collect inspirational quotes, and read/listen to inspirational books. God's inspiration is everywhere. He is rooting for you and wants to help set your goals on fire.

Time-Based and Measurable

Setting a specific date to reach a goal will make all the difference in your progress. Allotting yourself three months rather than leaving the completion date of your goals open-ended gives you something more tangible to work toward. We don't want to rush our fitness, but if we don't concern ourselves at all with the timeline of reaching our goals, then we may keep putting if off.

Along those lines, we also need to be tracking our progress in a quantifiable way because we're more likely to continue working toward our goals when we can see the difference being made. A food diary or an exercise journal is a great way to see how far we've come (perhaps losing two inches in our waist even though the scale shows just a few pounds of weight loss or going from never working out at all to getting daily exercise).

- Choose a method for tracking your progress. This can be as simple as a hand-written journal to document meals, measurements, body fat, scale weight, and daily exercise, or as detailed as an online app or band. These options provide specific details regarding caloric intake and expenditure. The Jawbone Up band, Argus, and Fitbit One are just a few examples.
- Select a regular day of the week to check your scale weight, body fat, and measurements. Body fat can be measured on a body composition scale, hand held body fat monitor, or with body-fat calibers. All of these products are available for purchase online. Measurements should be taken with an old-fashioned measuring tape in the exact same places: your upper arm, bellybutton, thighs, and hips. Taking measurements is very important because scale weight may not always show the

progress you have made. Take pictures once a month in the same outfit and stance to visibly see results.

- Circle a goal-completion date on your calendar. Twelve weeks is a realistic amount of time to start seeing results. Put calendar alerts in your phone to help remind you.
- Plan something special on your goal-completion date to celebrate your accomplishment and use it as motivation along the way.

Healthy

It's not a healthy goal to try to lose twenty pounds in a week or be able to run a full marathon without training for it months in advance. Healthy and realistic goals include weight loss of one to two pounds per week, lowering your blood pressure or cholesterol, and/or running two miles in under twenty minutes. Make sure your goal is setting you up for success.

- Is your goal realistic? Your goal should be achievable; this enables you to place healthy expectations on yourself.
- Make sure your goal is balanced and not extreme. No skipping meals, excessive exercise, or negative talk about yourself.
- Make sure to have a physical before beginning any new exercise program. A baseline blood profile is important in ruling out any underlying health issues, such as hypothyroidism, which can make weight loss almost impossible. Know your blood pressure and resting heart rate, and see if you can make these numbers go down as you become more physically fit.
- Practice appreciating your body for how it takes care of you rather than for what it looks like. Don't focus solely on your appearance when it comes to setting goals. Your body is your

vehicle, and its function goes far beyond its outer appearance. Consider how it carries you up the stairs, protects your vital organs, and enables you to experience each of your senses.

STOP WISHING, START DOING

Now faith is the substance of things hoped for, the evidence of things not seen.

—Hebrews 11:1 KJV

Once I realized that losing weight would require a lifestyle change, I needed the strength to be real with myself. I could no longer believe in a quick fix from a diet, but I couldn't rely on one from God either. Asking God to give me the strength against the things that kept me from lasting change helped me turn from wishing to goal setting.

If our goals do not follow the F.A.I.T.H. formula, then it might be safe to assume they're not goals at all. Consider the difference between a wish and a goal.

Wish: I want to lose ten pounds.
Goal: My goal is to lose ten pounds in order to feel more confident and have more energy when I'm playing with my children. I will accomplish this by working out five days a week for thirty minutes to an hour. I will eat five mini meals a day consisting of God-made, not man-made, foods. I will weigh myself every Wednesday and record my measurements. I'm committed to spending time in the Word of God every day—keeping my mind focused on who I am in the Word and not in the world. I will enjoy eating one meal of whatever I want on Sunday, but I will stick to the 5 Ps—Pause, Pray, Portion, Practice and Plan (covered in Step 7).

Can you see the difference? A goal clearly shows what's required of you to attain your desired outcome, and a wish is just talk.

It's in the day-to-day grind that we get lost in the shuffle of life. Having F.A.I.T.H. goals specifically lays out our daily responsibilities and takes all the guesswork out of how we will get there. Still, knowing what we need to do doesn't mean it will always get done. Staying close to God along this journey and seeking our daily strength through His Word ensures that we will experience a true lifestyle change and not treat this journey as we would a quick-fix diet program.

"BRING IT" TO GOD

Do not be anxious about anything, but in every situation, by prayer and petition, with thanksgiving, present your requests to God.

—Philippians 4:6 NIV

Working with my client Michelle was an adventure. Admittedly addicted to sugar and busy with two kids and a full-time job, she couldn't see how it was possible to get fit and healthy after failing to keep her weight down on countless fad diets. Receiving a report from her doctor, which warned her that she was at high risk for diabetes, had finally made her confront her lifestyle and choose to work with me. Still, she was uncertain about whether or not she could change.

Michelle had an all or nothing personality. She was in one day and out the next, so I knew only God could help her find balance. And, although she was a Christian, she had never considered asking God to join her on the journey to wellness. The notion actually surprised her, but she agreed to begin addressing personal issues in her F.I.T. Power Hour.

Bringing all the stress of her responsibilities, concern for her health, and uncertainty about whether she could change before God, Michelle was able to work through old hurts that she didn't realize were still affecting her.

Working with Michelle for over three months, I watched her transform from the inside out once she got her faith involved. She was able to explain that she had been turning to sugar for energy, but bringing her addiction to God helped her realize that it was actually making her energy crash and was giving her horrible headaches. With this new understanding of the role her vice was really playing in her life, it was easier for Michelle to minimize her intake of it.

Michelle and I worked on replacing her sugar fix with healthier alternatives that would sustain her energy. Feeling so much better made her officially kick the addiction, and realizing that her all-or-nothing mentality was extreme and that healthy is a lifestyle and not a race to the finish line also helped her to not feel like a failure and gave her the drive she needed to keep going.

Losing over twenty pounds to reduce her risk of diabetes was Michelle's physical goal, but she has since told me the biggest change came from the inside. She squared away in her mind that she wasn't going to turn to sugar to deal with her emotions any longer, and though she occasionally found herself reaching for that candy bar, she wasn't going to give up on herself, because God had shown her she could get healthy for good!

Taking this trip toward a healthier you is not a straight line. There certainly were plenty of bumps along the road for Michelle. Just as she did, you will have flat tires—bad days and moments when you just want to give up. But that's when you have to "Bring It!" Whatever you've got—from excuses to enthusiasm, bring it to God on a daily basis. On especially tough days of sadness, pain, or frustration, give it all to Him because if you don't bring it, He can't bless it.

He's cheering you on. He wants to help. You're not alone in this.

Spend your F.I.T. Power Hour working on your F.A.I.T.H. goals with God. If you only have twenty minutes here or there, He'll take them. When we "bring it" to God—whether that be our troubles or our very best, we find comfort and strength in Him to remain diligent in our faith and fitness.

Sometimes I have nothing to give, but I still give it to God. On these days, I usually end up having a great workout. The minute I hear "You're an Overcomer" or another encouraging, Christian song blasting through my headphones, the whole world feels better and I'm reminded that His strength is sufficient even on my weakest days. In this moment, I experience joy like no other.

Plug In to Your Power Source

My people are destroyed for lack of knowledge.
—Hosea 4:6 NASB

When we bring our weaknesses to God, He blesses us with His strength and power. Knowing we have access to that power allows us to turn saying into doing. Your best for the day is good enough when you're plugged in to God because He can do infinitely more through you than you could ever imagine on your own.

Know the power you have in God, and walk this health journey with Him. He is the best partner in success you'll ever find. He gives strength to the weak. (Isaiah 40:29) He gives beauty for ashes. (Isaiah 61:3) He gives us all we need for life and godliness. (2 Peter 1:3) He gives us grace to stand against the desires of our flesh. (James 4:6)

Don't make the mistake of thinking God is far away. When we're trying to get healthy, it can feel like a lonely battle, but He will be there with you if you invite Him. Spend time with Him, collect scriptures, and pray His Word back to Him in faith. At this point, we can't leave faith out of fitness and expect success.

GET F.I.T.

We personalize our F.I.T. Power Hour by creating F.A.I.T.H. goals to maximize our success. Learning the difference between a wish and a goal, we understand how to take words and turn them into action and then reality. Knowing our journey to health is not a straight line and committing to "Bring It" to God no matter what, He gives us the strength to deal with any frustrations, setbacks, or crummy days. Even if it's just twenty minutes, we know He'll take any time we bring Him and bless it. In Him we combine our faith with our fitness and get healthy through His power, not our own. He is our power source, and we need to be plugged in.

Reflection Questions:

- What are your F.A.I.T.H. goals?

  ____

  ____

  ____

- What are some setbacks that might occur? (They might be the very things that have hindered you in the past.)

  ____

  ____

  ____

Once your goals are well thought out and written down, they need to be put into practice. When you can see yourself doing something new, and figure out how to make it work in your daily life, then that practice becomes your reality. Let's go a step deeper and connect your physical goals with the right thinking.

- List three reasons why you will succeed this time. (What are

your lasting goals?)
- Why haven't you achieved these goals in the past?
- How are you going to overcome them?
- What are you going to do when you feel like giving up?
- Are you committed to stop wishing and start doing?

Here are a few ideas for how you can stop wishing and start doing today:

- Download the Bible onto your iPod and listen to it in the car.
- Collect three scriptures that you will pray over your health.
- Put some great Christian music on your iPod, upbeat songs you can work out to.
- Start your day with God (even if it's only one verse a day).
- Take a group exercise class with a friend.
- Write down your F.A.I.T.H. Goals in your journal and commit to your F.I.T. Power Hour.
- Write down the answers to the questions above and keep them where they won't be forgotten or lost.
- Whatever emotional state you find yourself in, "Bring It" to God!
- Tuck yourself in with a prayer of gratitude to God for all He does for you.

It isn't just one large change that leads to your success; it's all the daily decisions you make that turn dreaming into doing.

Our success is brought about through the daily decisions we make, and good decisions are easier to make when they are set in faith and clearly defined.

STEP SIX | EAT GOD-MADE, NOT MAN-MADE FOOD

Make Healthy Easy

> **Be well balanced (temperate, sober of mind), be vigilant *and* cautious at all times; for that enemy of yours, the devil, roams around like a lion roaring [in fierce hunger], seeking someone to seize upon *and* devour.**
>
> **—1 Peter 5:8 AMP**

This scripture instructs us to be balanced and shows us that we have a very real enemy that will seize the opportunity to destroy us when we aren't. Because many of us use food to cope with stress, we find ourselves mindlessly eating quite often. And although this coping mechanism may seem harmless, it can shake the foundation of health that we are trying to build into our lives. Balance means we are in control of our food choices, not controlled by them. Therefore, if you can't fill up on certain foods, you should question their value and their place in your diet.

Karen, or the "carb queen" (as she called herself), was a client of mine who longed and looked forward to diving into a bag of potato chips almost every day. One day as she was sharing her love of chips with me, she mentioned how odd it was that she could never seem to get full on them and that her cravings were insatiable.

Seeing an opportunity to explain the difference between God-made and man-made food, I asked Karen to consider why she was never fully satisfied with eating potato chips. If she wouldn't eat a whole bag of grapes or an endless amount of chicken salad, why was it that she couldn't feel full devouring a bag of chips?

When Karen couldn't answer my question, I shared with her that highly-processed man-made foods are so addicting that they stimulate brain activity similar to that of certain drugs. In addition, I explained how empty calories found in foods like potato chips don't provide the body with any nutrients to satisfy hunger, which was why she was still hungry after eating chips.

I went on to explain how consuming excess amounts of empty calories can turn into a vicious cycle of weight gain. Then I gave her a sample week of God-made meals. After only one week, Karen said she felt like a completely different person. She shared with me that eating God-made foods cleared her mind, increased her energy, and made her feel so much better.

IT MATTERS WHAT YOU EAT

> **Here I am! I stand at the door and knock. If anyone hears my voice and opens the door, I will come in and eat with that person, and they with me.**
>
> **—Revelation 3:20 NIV**

Have you invited God into your kitchen? This may seem like a new concept, but if we're going to be eating *God*-made foods, shouldn't God be involved? As we learn more about how to go about eating healthfully, it's important to remember that we're not doing this alone. We spend time with God during our F.I.T. Power Hour, but don't you think he would enjoy sitting down to eat with us too?

As we gain understanding about health and fitness God's way, I believe it will become more and more clear that He desires we eat to live, not live to eat. I don't mean we should not appreciate or even enjoy the food that He provides, but maybe there is a reason God-made food is not the food that we tend to overindulge in or become addicted to.

Perhaps there is a reason certain foods are found in nature and certain foods are not. If you think about it, eating an apple is much simpler than mixing together a batch of muffins for breakfast. And when you consider the health benefits of an apple, full of vitamins and nutrients, compared to a muffin, full of sugar and fat, it's a wonder why we don't always choose the apple.

Clearly taste plays a huge part in our daily food choices, but it is a fleeting sensation that leaves us seconds after each bite. Remember when we talked about finding lasting motivations for getting healthy? Well, that same rule applies to every meal we choose to partake of.

If we base our food choices on how "good" something tastes relative to a healthier alternative, then we are basing our decisions on something fleeting. This doesn't mean we must eat foods that we find distasteful; it means that, given the choice between a delicious, bacon-laden burger with fries we're sure to enjoy or a delicious Greek salad that will be equally satisfying (yet less guilt-ridden), we will invite God to eat with us and will choose God-made food.

Of course, God is not going to be offended if we choose a hamburger every now and then, but in doing so, are we eating to live or living to eat? Are we inviting God into our kitchens and worshiping Him with our food choices? Or are we hiding ourselves in our kitchens and worshiping the taste of the food we eat?

Are we eating to live or living to eat?

Last summer on vacation I was dying for a cupcake, so I ate one. Immediately, my head started spinning and my stomach felt sick. I wanted to remember how awful I felt after choosing to pursue taste over my lasting goals, so I pulled out my iPhone and took a video of myself explaining how I felt on the other side of choosing a craving over self-control. Let me tell you, it wasn't my best moment on camera.

Will you think about this the next time your impulses get the best of you? While there's nothing wrong with enjoying life, balance out how many times the cupcake wins and carefully consider if you ever feel better after eating a bunch of junk food.

MAKING SENSE OF NUTRITION

It has been argued that if we just eat less and move more, then we will be healthy, happy, and fit, but I don't buy it. It's true, we might lose some weight, but this method assumes health and fitness is merely a matter of calories, however, not all calories are created equal.

For example, if you allotted yourself 500 calories for a meal, you could either have chips and soda or salmon, salad, *and* a small sweet potato. I don't know about you, but the second meal sounds both more filling and more healthful than the first. Another thing to consider is that the bodies these two meals will produce are extremely different. If you want to produce a healthy and fit body, then remember a calorie is not just a calorie.

I brought up the term *macronutrients* in Step 1, but now let's look more closely at the major players in our diets.

Carbohydrates

Carbohydrates have a very bad reputation. Most people think of carbs as the enemy, but they are essential for producing energy and building muscle. Even God has a recipe for bread in the Bible: "And you, take wheat and barley, beans and lentils, millet and emmer, and put them into a single vessel and make your bread from them. During the number of days that you lie on your side, 390 days, you shall eat it." (Ezekiel 4:9 ESV)

Carbs are similar to calories in the sense that not all are created equally. For example, Ezekiel Bread is radically different than its white-bread counterparts. Comparing the ingredients of the two reveals the extreme difference between healthy, God-made carbs and processed carbs. Ezekiel bread contains complex, starchy, and fibrous carbohydrates, which are whole and unrefined. They are rich in fiber, satisfying, and healthful. Complex, God-made, carbohydrates are commonly found in whole plant foods and are typically high in vitamins and minerals.

Examples include:

- Green vegetables
- Whole grains and foods made from them, such as oatmeal, whole-grain pasta, and whole-grain breads
- Starchy vegetables, such as potatoes, sweet potatoes, and corn
- Beans, lentils, and peas

White breads, on the other hand, contain man-made, simple carbohydrates that are processed and refined products full of sugar. They're the foods you can't seem to get full on, and they are very low in fiber.

Examples include:

- White-flour bread and pasta
- Packaged chips, cookies, and cereals
- Jams and jelly
- Table sugar
- Candy
- Sodas

Refined carbohydrates are one of the main reasons Americans battle obesity. Any of these carbohydrates that aren't burned get stored as body fat. Therefore, our goal is to limit our intake of these foods and choose better sources of nutrition because, while eating processed foods every now and then won't kill us, living on them for long periods of time might cause us to become simultaneously malnourished and overweight.[7]

10 Reasons to Avoid Man-Made Carbs

1. They increase body fat.
2. They are full of empty calories—causing hunger even after a meal.
3. They raise LDL (bad) cholesterol.
4. They suppress our immune systems.
5. They are full of chemicals that our bodies were not made to digest.
6. They are the leading cause of obesity.
7. They raise the risk of diabetes.
8. They are addicting.
9. They are linked to depression and fatigue.
10. They alter our taste buds and make healthy foods less appetizing.

Protein

Made up of amino acids arranged in different combinations, protein is in all cell bodies and is a vital building block in the growth, maintenance, and repair of body tissues. Next to water, it is the most abundant substance in the human body.

Protein is an essential component to a balanced diet. However, carefully consider your protein sources. A hot dog is protein, but it's man-made. The more we choose God-made foods, the healthier we will be.

God-made protein sources include:

- Seafood

- Skinless chicken and turkey
- Lean beef (including tenderloin, sirloin, and eye of round)
- Eggs
- Low-fat or fat-free dairy products
- Lean pork (tenderloin)
- Beans

Protein preserves energy-burning muscle tissue and boosts energy expenditure because of two key characteristics: protein digestion and metabolism. These two processes require much energy and therefore burn more calories. It's a win-win situation because more energy is required to digest and metabolize protein while protein-rich foods keep us feeling full longer than carbohydrate-laden foods—reducing our urge to consume more calories and burning off the ones we have already consumed.[8]

Fats

People often think eating fat will make them fat, so they avoid it. But some fats are essential to our health. In fact, fat plays an important role in energy production, it satiates our appetites, and it makes our hair and skin look healthy and smooth. Including healthy fats in our diet can reduce the risk of diseases—diabetes, heart disease, obesity—and improve cholesterol levels. Like carbohydrates, there are different types of fats and some are better than others.

Monounsaturated and Polyunsaturated Fatty Acids

These types of fats can actually lower blood pressure, cholesterol, and the risk of heart disease.

Sources include:

- nuts
- avocados
- olive oil
- fatty fish (such as salmon)
- walnuts
- flax seeds

Saturated Fat

Saturated fats are known for raising cholesterol, so enjoy them infrequently or find healthy alternatives (a turkey burger versus a hamburger or homemade sweet potato fries versus French fries from a drive-through).

Sources include:

- meat
- dairy products (such as cheese, butter, and milk)

With our goal being a healthy heart, we should enjoy saturated fats in moderation. We don't need to eat pizza and hamburgers every day, but there's nothing wrong with having them occasionally, especially if we make our own healthy versions.

Trans fat

Doctors consider trans fat to be the worst, as it raises both LDL (bad cholesterol) and HDL (good cholesterol). Steer clear of the center aisles of the grocery store, which contain products loaded with trans fat.

Sources include:

- packaged crackers, cookies, and muffins
- anything battered or fried
- cakes and pies

- margarine and shortening
- non-dairy coffee creamers
- canned chili
- pre-packaged frozen meals

Sugar

Sugar is carefully hidden on many labels, and it doesn't have any nutritional value. While there's nothing wrong with occasionally enjoying ice cream or cookies, we need to retrain our taste buds to desire God's naturally sweet foods, such as fruit.

Here is a list of some of the different names of sugar to help you know what to look for on labels:

- **Syrup (such as high-fructose corn syrup)**
- **Caramel**
- **Molasses**
- **Fructose (natural sugar from fruits)**
- **Lactose (natural sugar from milk)**
- **Sucrose (common table sugar; made from fructose and glucose)**
- **Maltose (sugar made from grain)**
- **Glucose (natural sugar, product of photosynthesis)**
- **Dextrose (a form of glucose)**

An especially compelling reason to avoid sugar is that a great body of research shows it to possess addictive qualities with effects similar to certain drugs. One such study concluded that "intermittent access to sugar can lead to behavioral and neurochemical changes that resemble the effects of a substance of abuse."[9] Have you ever noticed the addictive quality of your favorite sugary foods? Let's choose to enjoy these occasionally and in moderation, and let's find healthy alternatives because sugary foods are full of empty calories and they alter our taste buds to find naturally sweetened foods less satisfying.

Substituting your favorite treats is as simple as exchanging flours and sweeteners and trans fat oils for their healthier counterparts. For instance, try making a healthy apple pie with almond flour, coconut oil, and honey or my favorite no-bake energy bites with dark chocolate chips, natural peanut butter, honey, and whey protein powder to satisfy a sweet tooth.

When it comes to the amount of sugar we should (or shouldn't) be consuming, The World Health Organization suggests making it only five percent of our daily caloric intake. For most women this is approximately six teaspoons a day (about three granola bars or one cup of yogurt), as opposed to the twenty-two teaspoons most Americans consume on a daily basis.[10]

Because most of us are used to consuming so much sugar, you may need to set your goal slightly higher than five percent, especially if six teaspoons seems overwhelmingly small in comparison to your normal intake. However, keep working to make that number drop. You won't regret the difference you feel in your energy or the success you experience in your health goals.

IT MATTERS WHAT YOU DRINK

Food selection is not the only thing we need to keep in mind when considering God-made versus man-made and sugar intake. Rarely do we consider our beverage choices, but sugar we consume from a convenience store soda in one place and a latte from a drive-through somewhere else may accumulate exponentially over the course of one day. For instance, each eight-ounce serving of a bottled iced tea contains twenty-three grams of sugar, and lemonade and soda each have twenty-seven grams.

I think people get lost in the math, but twenty-seven grams of sugar is roughly seven teaspoons. Imagine pouring seven teaspoons of sugar into your drink—and this is just in one eight-ounce serving! Most drinks are over sixteen ounces, so, from our example, they would include fourteen teaspoons of sugar, which equals 224 empty calories in just one beverage.

Try replacing fruit juices, sodas, and sugary coffee beverages with hot tea from an assortment of tea bags. There are so many delicious flavors, from citrus to blackberry mojito to strawberry lemonade. Also try sparkling water with your favorite fruit slices, or stick with plain water.

Now that we have educated ourselves in spite of all the confusion surrounding what to eat, let's be careful to avoid obsessing over our body image or practicing extreme dietary restrictions (unless medically advised). When our bodies become the major focus in our lives, we become our own idols, and this is sin. God should always be our focus. An obsession with weight loss can easily move into extreme behaviors and become anorexia, bulimia, or the opposite extreme, gluttony.

As I mentioned in Step 1, most diets play with macronutrient percentages by limiting protein, carbohydrates, or fat. This is a "one size fits all" approach, but we all have different body types and goals. For instance, a person trying to gain muscle would not require the same macronutrient split as one who just wants to lose fat. To gain muscle one should consume high protein and moderate to high starchy carbohydrates whereas to lose fat one would stick with moderate protein and low starchy carbohydrates, coming mostly from fibrous sources. Different goals require different menus, and no single strategy yields the same results for every body.

When I was training to be a fitness model, I would eat high protein, moderate good fats, high fibrous carbs, and low starchy carbs. My morning meal would consist of starchy carbs and the rest of the day I only consumed fibrous carbs from vegetable sources. Every three days I would add an additional starchy carbohydrate back into my diet—tricking my body and making it look leaner. This is called carbohydrate cycling and, though it is effective, the results are temporary. My body couldn't maintain the results unless I was willing to continue to eat that way.

So, don't buy the smoke and mirrors. Get healthy, love your body the way God made it, and fuel it in a way that supports what you want it to be able to do, not just what you want it to look like.

Here are some simple guidelines to consider when it comes to eating healthfully:

- **Don't try to "out-train" an unhealthy diet. Research shows that weight loss is 75% what we eat and only 25% exercise.[11]**
- **Avoid diets that adjust macronutrient splits. They may be beneficial if you are trying to add muscle or lose fat, but you must be consistent and committed to maintain the results.**
- **Find a balanced eating plan. You'll find long-term success when protein, fat, and carbs work together to make you feel more satisfied.**
- **Eat quality ingredients instead of stressing over exact quantities (i.e. calorie counting) and opting for pre-packaged snacks or frozen meals.**

MAKING A "GOD-MADE" PLATE

Everything is permissible for me, but not everything is helpful. Everything is permissible for me, but I will not allow anything to control me.... Therefore, glorify God with your bodies.

—1 Corinthians 6:12, 20b ISV

PROTEIN	STARCHY CARBS	FIBROUS CARBS	GOOD FATS	CONDIMENTS
3 ounces or the size of the palm of your hand	*1/2 cup or a rounded handful*	*1 cup or the size of your fist*	*1 tsp or index finger tip for cooking* *2 tbsp or thumb joint to tip for nut butters* *1/4 cup or 1 handful for nut servings*	*2 tbsp or thumb joint to tip*
Chicken Breast	Sweet Potato	Kale	Extra Virgin Olive Oil	Black Pepper, Lemon Pepper
Turkey Breast	White Potato	Broccoli	Coconut Oil	Salsa
Bison	Yam	Green Beans	Avocados & Avocado Oil	Stevia
Lean or Ground Beef	Whole-Grain Breads & Pastas	Bell Peppers, Any Color	Flaxseed Oil	Dry spices, Basil, Thyme, Oregano
Sirloin Steak or Ground	Ezekiel Bread, Tortillas, Muffins, Pocket Breads	Spinach & Any Leafy Greens	Walnut Oil	Mustard
Salmon	Legumes, Lentils, Peas, & Beans	Cucumbers	Macadamia Oil	Healthy Oil-Based Salad Dressing
Tilapia	Squash	Brussels Sprouts	Canola Oil	Balsamic/Apple Cider Vinegar
Tuna	Steel-cut Oats	Cauliflower	Sunflower Oil	Tabasco/Hot Sauces
Eggs	Bulgur	Onions	Sesame Oil	Garlic, Onion, Curry, Chili & Ginger Powder
Low-fat Cottage Cheese	Quinoa	Celery	Nuts	Lemon Wedges & Orange Slices
Greek Yogurt	Brown Rice/ Brown Rice Pasta	Mushrooms	Nut Butters	Cinnamon, Pumpkin Spices
High Quality Whey Protein Powder, Low Sugar	Whole-Grain, Low-Sugar Cereals	Asparagus	Seeds	Mrs. Dash Salt-Free & MSG Free Spices

In spite of all the macronutrient breakdowns and scientific ways we could go about analyzing what and how much we should eat, *F.I.T.* eating is designed to be simple. God gave us everything we need to get healthy. Not only has he provided a plethora of healthy foods to choose from, He even gave us our two hands to measure with.

God-made food is not limiting, as there is a bounty of God-made foods available to us. A God-made plate includes a portion of lean protein, a God-made carbohydrate, and a healthy fat. Below are some examples of what a God-made plate might look like throughout the day.

Breakfast: Hard-boiled eggs, steel-cut oats with flax seed and cinnamon.

Lunch: Chicken breast with a small sweet potato and green beans with a drizzle of olive oil.

Dinner: Salmon (protein and good fat) with quinoa and a kale salad.

Snacks: Apples and nut butter, Greek yogurt and berries, or half of an Ezekiel tortilla wrap with turkey, avocado, romaine lettuce, and mustard.

You can find more meal options at the end of this chapter, after the Get F.I.T. section or online at www.kimdolanleto.com.

The F.I.T. Hand Chart

The F.I.T. Hand Chart (on page 96) shows how our hands are natural measuring utensils for our daily meals. Sometimes weighing and portioning exact quantities of our carbohydrate, protein, and fat sources seems like overkill. Because we're ditching diets, I think it's important to find an easy, no-fuss way to know how much we should be eating. The hand chart is the best tool I have found to portion food without becoming preoccupied. Let it be a reference as you learn to prepare a God-made plate.

Don't overthink food and underestimate yourself. God-made eating is balanced. There are no extremes, pills, guilt, or quick fixes here. Eating a slice of pizza or a candy bar does not make you a failure because we all fail our way to success. And when we fall, we get back up faster, and we don't let food or our flesh control us. The Lord is by our side—holding our hands so we won't give up, and His spirit is alive in us.

Don't over think food and underestimate yourself!

HAND SYMBOL	EQUIVALENT	FOODS	CALORIES
	Fist 1 cup	Rice Pasta Fruit Veggies	200 200 75 40
	Palm 3 ounces	Meat Fish Poultry	160 160 160
	Handful 1/2 cup	Nuts Raisins	170 85
	2 Handfuls 1 cup	Chips Popcorn Pretzels	150 120 100
	Thumb 1 ounce	Peanut Butter Hard Cheese	170 100
	Thumb Tip 1 teaspoon	Cooking Oil Mayonnaise Butter Sugar	40 40 35 15

GET F.I.T.

When it comes to eating healthfully, remember Keep It Simple Sister (K.I.S.S.). Don't overthink it. Eat God-made, balanced meals every three to four hours along with healthy, balanced snacks in between. Don't skip meals and don't get caught up in the deprivation-overconsumption cycle of dieting. Start off making small changes and let small successes build over time to show you what you're capable of. Make God your partner and you'll find the winning routine that will make your new lifestyle sustainable and your results lasting.

Reflection Questions:

- What are some God-made foods you really enjoy? What man-made foods could you swap out with these healthier treats?

  ____

  ____

  ____

- How will you make your meal plan sustainable?

  ____

  ____

  ____

Follow the strategies below to begin implementing F.I.T. eating into your life.

Strategy #1: Don't Skip Meals. Frequently skipping meals will cause your body to go into starvation mode. It will hold on to fat rather than burn it. Eating regular meals and snacks keeps your energy up, your blood sugar consistent, and your metabolism working.

Strategy #2: Plan meals and cook in advance. Cook on Sundays and freeze your food. Preparing meat ahead of time, baking sweet potatoes, steaming rice, making whole grain pasta, and chopping veggies and fruit will give you more time and make F.I.T. eating easy.

Strategy #3: Stay hydrated and avoid hidden calories. Make sure you're adequately hydrated. Our bodies are 60 percent water, so even mild dehydration can drain our energy and make us feel tired. Aim for a minimum of eight glasses of water per day.

Strategy #4: Commit to small changes and see BIG results. Do you think F.I.T. eating equates to radically changing your diet and giving up all your favorite foods? That's not the case. Make changes gradually and beware of the "all or nothing" mentality. If you're struggling with changing your lifestyle, commit to one thing at a time. Begin with your beverage selections, then add in more veggies with your meals, and then tackle your kitchen and cooking. Getting healthy is a process, not a one-time event. Take it step by step.

Strategy #5: Learn basic alternatives. **(See chart on next page.)**

F.I.T. FOODS

Eat This, Not That

- Ezekiel or Whole-grain bread
- All-natural nut butter
- Stevia or Honey
- Skim, almond, or coconut milk
- Low-fat cheese
- Lean turkey, chicken, or beef
- Broiled, baked, or steamed
- Spaghetti squash or brown rice
- Sweet potatoes
- Fresh vegetables
- Fresh fruit
- Oatmeal
- Greek yogurt
- Olive oil
- Dark chocolate and berries
- Whole-grain pizza crust
- Baked apples with cinnamon
- Fat-free frozen yogurt
- Air-popped popcorn
- Hummus or avocado
- Homemade, whole-grain bread crumbs
- Mineral water (flavored or plain)
- Coffee with stevia
- Iced tea with lemon or orange slices

- White bread
- Processed nut butters
- Un-natural sweeteners
- Whole milk
- Full-fat cheese
- High-fat meats
- Fried or breaded foods
- Processed pasta or rice
- Regular potatoes
- Canned vegetables
- Canned fruit
- High-sugar cereals
- Sour cream
- Vegetable oil
- Candy bar
- Regular pizza crust
- Cookies
- Ice cream
- Potato chips
- Mayonnaise
- Processed bread crumbs
- Soda pop (diet or regular)
- Coffee with full-fat cream and sugar
- Bottled, artificially sweetened iced teas

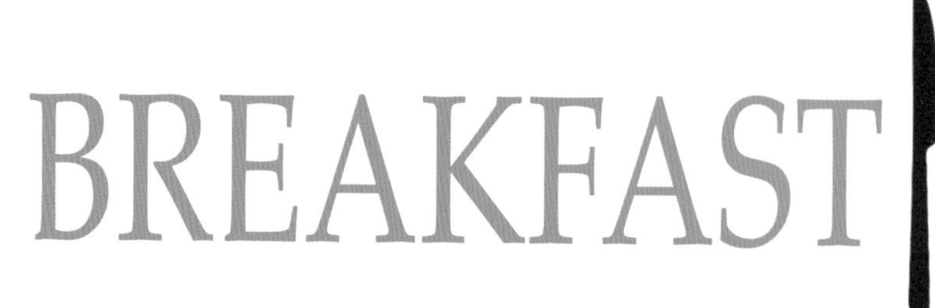

PROTEIN + STARCH + FRUIT + GOOD FAT

- **Whole-grain or Ezekiel toast with almond butter and apple slices**
- **Ezekiel pocket bread filled with 2 scrambled eggs (or 4 egg whites and one yolk), mushrooms, and peppers**
- **Whole-grain toast with Greek yogurt, pistachios, and a drizzle of honey**
- **Oatmeal sweetened with black cherry concentrate and sprinkled with walnuts**
- **Greek yogurt with raspberries and chia seeds**
- **Smoothie:** handful of spinach + frozen berries (or fruit of choice) + ¼ avocado (sounds weird, but makes for a creamy texture while adding good fat) + ½ cup water or almond or coconut milk + 1 scoop vanilla protein powder
- **Protein shake and raspberries**
- **Protein pancake + 1 tbs nut butter**
- **Egg bake + slice avocado + fruit:** throw a dozen eggs in a bowl, mix, add lots of veggies and a little feta cheese, pour into 9x13" pan and bake at 350 degrees until golden brown
- **Chia seed pudding + fruit**
- **Cottage cheese + fruit**

LUNCH

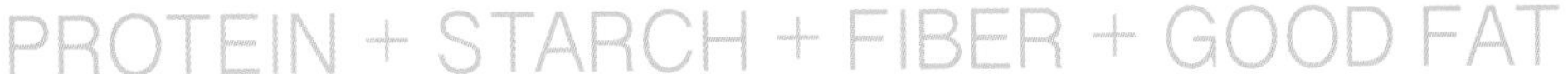

- **Lean protein + ½ cup brown rice or small sweet potato + 1 cup veggies + drizzle of olive oil**
- **Chili:** cook lean ground beef, chicken, or turkey, beans, tomatoes, any other veggies you'd like together in large pot on stove for 45 minutes to an hour + side salad with veggies and balsamic vinegar and olive oil
- **Chicken or steak (lean) fajita meat + peppers + onions + ½ cup brown rice + lettuce + ½ an avocado + salsa**
- **Healthy pizza:** use whole-grain pita or flat bread and add sauce, lean protein, veggies, and a light amount of fresh mozzarella, bake at 350 degrees until cooked through
- **Spaghetti:** 1 cup (cooked) brown rice pasta + low-sugar spaghetti sauce + lean ground turkey, chicken, or beef + side salad with veggies and balsamic vinaigrette
- **Turkey burger + green beans or veggie of choice + ½ cup squash or 1 small sweet potato**
- **Taco salad:** lean ground meat + lettuce + peppers + ½ an avocado (Make the taco salad into a taco bowl by adding ½ cup of brown rice)
- **Build your own salad:** Big bowl of greens + lean protein + veggies + olive oil and garlic dressing + ½ cup of butternut squash soup

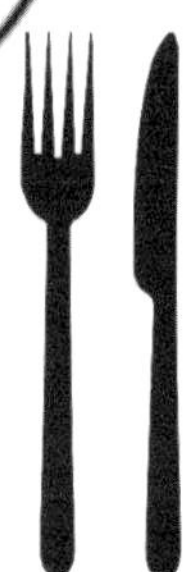

DINNER

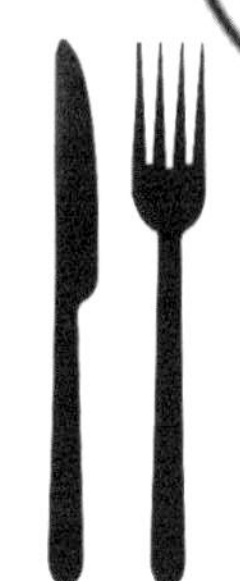

PROTEIN + STARCH + FIBER + GOOD FAT

- **Salmon (protein and good fat) with quinoa and a kale salad**
- **4 oz. chicken + 1-2 cup veggies (broccoli, cauliflower) + couscous**
- **Spaghetti squash + 1 cup spaghetti sauce with lean protein (ground chicken or lean ground beef) + side salad and balsamic vinegar and olive oil**
- **Taco salad:** lean ground meat + lettuce + tomatoes + peppers + ½ avocado
- **Chicken fajitas + peppers + onions + lettuce + ½ an avocado + salsa**
- **Stuffed peppers:** stuff pepper with lean ground turkey, chicken, or beef and veggies, bake at 400 degrees until pepper is soft
- **Breakfast omelet for dinner:** 2 eggs (or 4 egg whites + 1 yolk) made your way + spinach + peppers + mushrooms + sprinkle of feta cheese
- **Lean flank steak + roasted zucchini + green beans + drizzle of olive or sesame oil**
- **Build your own salad:** Big bowl of greens + lean protein + veggies + olive oil and garlic dressing + handful of sunflower or pumpkin seeds

SNACKS

PROTEIN + GOOD FAT AND/OR CARB

- Raw veggies + dip (use your favorite creamy dressing, but only use 1 tbs and mix with 2 tbs of Greek yogurt for less fat and calories)
- Apple with walnuts or nut butter (measured)
- Greek yogurt with berries (my favorite!)
- Oatmeal with flavored protein powder (1 scoop)
- Tuna with whole-grain crackers
- Non-Fat Cottage cheese + fruit of choice
- Romaine lettuce turkey wrap + a little mustard
- Small, whole-grain pita with 1 slice of cheese and 1 tbs of low-sodium tomato sauce and fresh garlic and basil (another favorite)
- Leftover chicken and fruit kabob (my daughter's favorite)
- Ezekiel bread with nut butter (for those days when you're really hungry)
- Brown rice cake with nut butter
- 1 or 2 Hard-boiled eggs + veggie slices of choice
- Small banana + chocolate protein shake

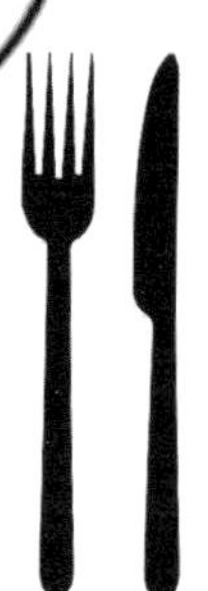

DESSERT

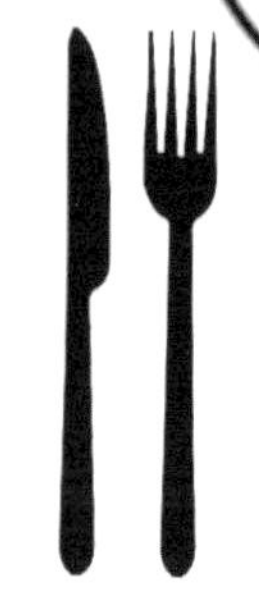

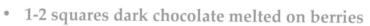

- **1-2 squares dark chocolate melted on berries**
- **Chia pudding (make with cocoa, almond, or coconut milk and berries for a sweet treat)**
- **Baked apple or pear:** Bake an apple or pear drizzled with honey and/or stevia and sprinkled with cinnamon at 425 degrees for about 30 minutes
- **Frozen yogurt bites:** Mix you're favorite sweet topping (nut butter, cocoa, vanilla, or stevia) with Greek yogurt, dollop into an ice-cube tray, and freeze. (When ready, enjoy 3-4. Or do 2-3 and dip in 1 square of chocolate.)
- **Treat-like yogurt:** You can also do the above un-frozen for a normal yogurt serving size.
- **Protein pudding:** 1 scoop flavored protein powder + almond or coconut milk or water (mixed to desired consistency)
- **Banana ice cream:** Take 1½ frozen bananas, ⅓ cup almond or coconut milk, ¼ cup 0% Greek yogurt, and 1 tsp of honey, and blend in food processor. (Makes one serving.)
- **No-Bake Energy Bites:** Mix 1 cup (dry) oatmeal, ½ cup chocolate chips, ½ cup peanut butter, ½ cup ground flaxseed, ⅓ cup honey, 1 tsp vanilla. Roll into balls. Refrigerate and enjoy! (Makes about 2 dozen balls.)

STEP SEVEN | CHOOSE SELF-CONTROL

Find Lasting Motivation and Implement the 5 Ps

For the moment all discipline seems painful rather than pleasant, but later it yields the peaceful fruit of righteousness to those who have been trained by it.
—Hebrews 12:11 ESV

After taking my daughter to school one morning, I went to Starbucks to get a green tea. As I walked by the tables, I couldn't help but notice cinnamon roles, lemon cake, and all the frappuccinos and lattes. When I got in my car, I sat there for a moment and thought, *Hey, that's not fair. I want to eat all those treats too. Why do I have to go without that stuff?* I was mad, and that's when the self-justification attacked: *I deserve to eat whatever I want. After all, it's just one meal, and I've been so good for so long. You only live once, right?*

In that moment I was tempted to give up. But, after I put the key in the ignition and started my car, the song "No Turning Back" by Israel Houghton and New Breed blasted through the speakers and into my thoughts. Immediately I felt convicted and remembered my "Why," my motivation. *I need to be healthy to be around for my daughter and to carry out the plans God has for me to the best of my ability.* And I wasn't turning back. I was committed to going forward with God.

How many times have you given up? Like a kid in a candy store, have you gone crazy enjoying all of your favorite foods and treats right before strategizing your next diet plan? It's easier to convince yourself that you will really get healthy for good after bingeing and experiencing that sickening feeling of guilt often associated with overeating. Planning your next diet after a plate of nachos or a second bowl of ice cream isn't healthy, and the shame that follows is not a motivation that lasts.

I've witnessed hundreds of people work tirelessly to lose weight only to gain it all back. In fact, more than 80% of people who have lost weight on a dieting plan regain all or more of it after two years.[12] Sadly, this is the very result of most diets because the common short-term mindset of dieting overrules the lifestyle change that should be happening. Lasting change requires lasting commitment.

I can't even count the number of times I've lost weight only to gain it all back. Until I got my mindset right, I was on a never-ending roller coaster of restriction and overconsumption—happiness and depression. A pivotal shift in my thinking came when I realized I wanted to be happy and healthy all the time, not only after I'd lost weight for a special occasion.

I realized that events such as high school reunions and summer vacations only provide motivation until they pass. After these temporary motivators ran their course, I didn't know where self-control was supposed to come from. In order to find lasting motivation, I had to realize that my roller coaster of dieting was getting me nowhere. I could be disciplined long enough to lose some weight, but I never addressed my bad habits or prayed for the strength to be free of them.

The 5 Ps

My husband suggested we get Mexican food one day after I received some bad news. I knew he was trying to cheer me up, and chips and salsa are my kryptonite, so I agreed. After being seated at the restaurant and eating several chips, I realized I hadn't prayed over the food or over the bad news I had received earlier. Instead of turning to God,

I turned to food to anesthetize me through the pain of my bad day. We stopped eating, said a prayer, and I felt a little Godly nudge to put on the spirit of self-control. Between pausing and praying, everything changed.

The enemy of self-control is instant gratification; it's that one cheesy nacho that leads to a whole plate more. Keep in mind that you're not a failure because of what you eat—enjoy a treat every now and then; but, just as we need balance when eating healthfully, we need to balance our moments of indulgence as well. One way we might do so is by implementing the 5 Ps, which help us to keep our focus on God and free of the tendency to overeat.

The enemy of self-control is instant gratification.

Practice these 5 Ps at every meal:

1. **Pause** before you decide to eat and ask yourself if you're really hungry or if you're just feeding your emotions, boredom, or stress.
2. **Pray** before meals. Ask God to help you eat the right foods in the right amounts and for the discipline to take care of your body (His temple). I pray to surrender my appetite to Him daily and remind myself using the acronym S.A.F.E. (Surrender Appetite Faithfully Every Day).
3. **Portion** each meal. Be mindful of the amount of food you're eating. If you want to indulge in a treat, serve yourself a portion on a plate and then put the rest away. Refrain from eating out of containers, bags, boxes, or pans.
4. **Practice** eating slowly. Take smaller bites and chew them between ten to twenty times. Try setting your fork down between bites and thinking of food as fuel and nourishment rather than comfort or reward.
5. **Plan** ahead. Make healthy meals as often as you can and always have healthy snacks on hand. Don't wait until you're hungry to find food. I know I rarely make good choices when I am starving.

MOTIVATION THAT LASTS

You are the light of the world. A city set on a hill cannot be hidden. Nor do people light a lamp and put it under a basket, but on a stand, and it gives light to all in the house. In the same way, let your light shine before others, so that they may see your good works and give glory to your Father who is in heaven.

—Matthew 5:14-16 ESV

A Healthy Body Glorifies God

The Faith Inspired Transformation is Christ-centered, not self-centered.

Let's be honest, being unhealthy and out of shape makes it harder for our light to shine. Putting aside what we look like physically, where are we going to get the energy and endurance we need to carry out our God-given purposes if we're overweight and out of shape? We need to find the motivation to get healthy, and we need to discipline ourselves to see its value because we each have a unique calling on our lives. Carrying out our purposes without our health makes this very difficult.

Our flesh will give up and quit on us every time, so we can't rely on our own strength—that's why the Faith Inspired Transformation is Christ-centered, not self-centered.

Don't cheat yourself and live your life feeling less than who God created you to be. Being unhealthy can do this to us. Getting healthy means you put away the excuses and ask God to help you seek health with the right motives. If you allow Him, He will let you know when you start heading down the wrong path.

If you've been unsuccessful getting healthy in the past, tell yourself this time is different and ask God for help. Believe in yourself because

He does! Making health your lifestyle and focusing your transformation on God is the right motivation. It will last because God is everlasting.

The following are examples of motivations that last and motivations that do not last. Measure your own motives against these two lists and consider whether it is enduring or fleeting.

Lasting Motivations:

- I want to be a healthy role model for my child.
- I want to avoid heart disease, diabetes, and obesity.
- I want the energy to play with my children/grandchildren without running out of breath.
- I want to feel good about myself and comfortable in my own skin.
- I don't want my weight to interfere with the vision God has for my life.
- I want to be confident for the right reasons.

I will satisfy you with a long life. I will show you how I will save you.

—Psalm 91:16 GWT

Motivation that doesn't last:

- I want to look good in a swimsuit.
- I want a six-pack.
- I want to make people jealous.
- I want to be in better shape than all my friends.
- I want to be popular or famous.

For the mind that is set on the flesh is hostile to God, for it does not submit to God's law; indeed, it cannot.

—Romans 8:7 ESV

FIND YOUR "WHY"

It was the phone call we all dread. I can still hear my mom on the other line—her voice was shaky and she could barely speak. I fell to my knees when she said, "You need to get to the hospital right away. Your dad had a stroke."

My dad was only forty-seven on that day which still haunts me. At that moment my life changed. I was thirty and unhealthy. Busy working all day in the pharmaceutical industry, my diet was awful and working out was something I had put off—excusing myself by believing I just didn't have the time.

Realizing that my dad would never be the same and watching him suffer from paralysis in his face and the entire left side of his body was my wake-up call. Sitting by his hospital bed, I vowed never to be in the same situation. And I meant it, but I had no idea where to begin to avoid it.

Researching how to eat healthfully and include exercise in my daily life was a struggle, but seeing my dad in such a debilitated state was a glaring reminder that I couldn't take health for granted. Around this time I had a blood profile test done and learned my cholesterol was high. It seemed I was on the same path as my dad. I needed to change, and I knew I couldn't do it alone.

Genetics are a frightening thing. Both of my grandfathers died young, one from a stroke and one from a combination of a heart attack and cancer. Most of my family struggles with their weight, and looking at my prospective future through them, I felt sad—like I had a death sentence looming over me. It seemed so unfair, but it changed me. I took my concerns to God and began practicing the 5 Ps.

Being terrified of heart disease motivates me to this day, but looking back on that time, I was so confused and insecure about how to get healthy. Thinking about how many times I had begun a diet and quit haunted me and made me feel like an absolute failure.

My change started on the inside. I had to change the way I thought about food, exercise, and my time. Truthfully, I wanted to believe what happened to my dad would never happen to me. But the thought that it could if I didn't work to proactively change it finally took over.

Changing my health and my habits was a long and arduous process. It seemed so much easier to put it off or give up and keep living the way I had been, but I thought of my dad and asked God to help me know what to do. Initially, I felt awkward asking God to give me the strength, knowledge, and determination to change my lifestyle. But the more prayers He answered, the more self-control I had.

I want to live without heart disease. I don't want to have a stroke at forty-seven and die of a heart attack at sixty-one as my father did. I want to be a strong and positive role model for my daughter and live a long, healthy, and active life so that I can accomplish the tasks God calls me to accomplish. My life-changing motivation was found in heartbreak. It was hard to see any purpose in the midst of watching my father struggle, but it gave me my "Why."

Have you ever had an experience similar to mine, where you thought, *How did this happen? How did I end up here?* Let's be honest, although the pounds seem to appear overnight, they've been a while in the making. So, what will motivate you to implement the 5 Ps and exercise self-control? Whatever it is, make sure your "Why" falls into one of the following categories:

- **Relational**—being there for your children or spouse.
- **Medical**—reducing your risk of disease and enabling your ability to live life to the fullest.
- **Spiritual**—living out the purposes God has for you and being available to think of and help others in need.

Getting healthy is a process, so my health transformation did not end with finding lasting motivators or implementing the 5 Ps during my meal times. This should not be the end for you either, but it is a good place to start if you are as lost as I was when I began. Don't give up on your goals because you don't immediately see an outward change. Find your lasting motivation and keep practicing the 5 Ps. Begin to see yourself transforming from the inside out with every healthy meal and workout.

GET F.I.T.

Seeking good health as a Godly lifestyle is what changes everything. Finding our "Why" makes us think twice when we want to grab man-made snacks at the office, overeat at every meal, or even skip our F.I.T Power Hour. It's that extra push that keeps us going when we feel like giving up.

Reflection Questions:

- What is your "Why," and how will it help you practice self-control in the future?

  ____

  ____

  ____

- Which of the 5 Ps do you struggle with most? How might implementing that particular step affect your self-control during a meal?

  ____

  ____

  ____

Try the following strategies to stay motivated on your F.I.T. journey.

Strategy #1: Keep your "Why" in view. Make an inspiration board with motivating scriptures, pictures, and inspirational quotes. Include The 5 Ps along with these eating and exercising acronyms: S.A.F.E (Surrender Appetite Faithfully Every day) and W.O.R.K. (Work It, Own it, Rock it, Kill it).

Strategy #2: Make a pact with God. Agree to honor Him with your health and recognize that you cannot do this alone.

GET F.I.T.

Strategy #3: Tell the world. Post your workouts on social networking sites or blog about your fitness journey. This is a great way to stay motivated and encourage other people at the same time. You have the ability to transform someone else's life. Isn't that a reason to keep going?

Strategy #4: Track progress and celebrate your success. Get the right tools. Fitness apps and a personal journal are tangible ways to track your progress and literally see yourself succeeding. Learn to reward yourself with something other than food. Pedicures, massages, and new fitness outfits or gear are little reminders that you are worth it.

Strategy #5: Take the F.I.T. Challenge. Go to kimdolanleto.com right now and sign up for the F.I.T. Challenge. Join a group of women who want to see you succeed. If you need recipes, workouts, scriptures, support, and motivation, you will find it here. Get in the loop with our F.I.T. Group and take your faith and fitness to another level.

STEP EIGHT | CHANGE YOUR PERSPECTIVE

Find Joy In Every Situation

So we fix our eyes not on what is seen, but on what is unseen, since what is seen is temporary, but what is unseen is eternal.

—2 Corinthians 4:18 NIV

It was 5 a.m. on a hot Arizona morning, and I had just begun my morning run. My body felt like an old car trying to start up. It was screaming at me and complaining with every step. A good ten minutes passed before everything kicked into gear and I felt warmed up.

On this particular day I was feeling sorry for myself. I was thinking about how I had to work out first thing in the morning or I wouldn't have another opportunity. I was irritated because my family would still be sleeping by the time I was done running, showering, making breakfast, and packing lunches. That seemed unfair and just irked me.

With the sun barely peeking over the mountains, and my mind in a state of utter turmoil, I could see a man running ahead of me with a stride that seemed off. I ran faster to make sure he was okay. As I drew nearer to him, I realized he had survived a stroke, as his body was paralyzed on his entire left side. My heart sank, and I felt as though God was sending me a message.

Remember my dad? His stroke was my life-changing reason to get healthy. So, this moment didn't seem to be a mere coincidence. I stopped the man who was running and said, "I have to applaud you.

You are truly amazing."

This man was in his early 80s, had survived a stroke, and was still running at five o'clock in the morning even though he had every reason not to be. I told him that I didn't feel like running that morning and had to force myself to do so. He responded by saying, "Well, at least we can."

His perspective filled my heart with gratitude. Oh, boy. He was right. It's all about perspective. After that encounter, my dreaded run felt more like a privilege, and I couldn't wait to get home and have breakfast made, lunches packed, and everything ready for my family when they woke up.

CONTROLLING EMOTIONS

The joy of the Lord is your strength.
—Nehemiah 8:10 NIV

In the book of Nehemiah, the Israelites (God's chosen people) were carried away into exile, but God preserved a remnant to stay in the Land of Israel. These people heard the Word of the Lord spoken to them by a prophet and realized that they had not been living according to God's commands. Filled with remorse and guilt and shame, the people began to weep and mourn over the bad choices they made in the past. In the midst of their mourning, the prophet Ezra told the people to turn from sorrow and to celebrate their new understanding of how they should be living because God set up such a system for their benefit.

You see, the Israelites understood their failures, but that wasn't enough to evoke real, lasting change in their lives. They needed to see beyond the negative emotions brought on by their realization and believe that God loved them and wanted to bless them despite what they did in the past. In short, they needed to see the situation from His point of view.

God celebrated the fact that His people recognized the wrong they did in the past and that their hearts were opened to the possibility of transformation. He wanted them to celebrate as well and to know that he was rooting for them.

Much like the Israelites, many of us have made mistakes or experienced hurt in the past that have since determined the ways in which we see and treat ourselves. Recognizing those mistakes and realizing that we have fallen short is a difficult pill to swallow, but accepting that the love of God washes away those mistakes should be the most transformative and joy-giving message we ever receive.

Perhaps we don't always understand, as the Israelites did, why we have to face challenging times. But, even when we can't recognize why we struggle, the answer is to settle our emotions and find the joy of the Lord in the midst of hardship.

If the joy of the Lord is our strength, then happiness isn't material; it's a choice we make in those tough moments to see Him working in our circumstances rather than focusing on our problems. I find joy by grabbing my daughter and hugging her, playing my favorite Christian song that makes me feel overwhelmed by God's love and His presence, choosing to see people through the eyes of grace—remembering all the things God has forgiven me of, and recognizing when I choose gratitude over complaining.

Even if you make mistakes along the way, don't let yourself be controlled by self-doubt, laziness, depression, or any other negative feeling along this F.I.T. journey. Let the joy of the Lord be your strength, and feel the difference it makes. For example, the next time you are dreading a cardio workout, think about your health from a different perspective. Take your focus off of how much you would rather sit on the couch and catch up on your favorite TV shows and consider your amazing heart, which beats approximately 100,000 times a day (That's over 36 million times a year!) and how it is strengthened when you exercise. Now that's perspective!

Happiness Is a Choice

I am convinced that life is 10% what happens to me and 90% of how I react to it. And so it is with you...we are in charge of our attitudes.

—Charles R. Swindoll

One night at a women's Bible study I lead, I went around the table asking my friends, "How do you define happiness?" Their answers were as follows:

- *Appreciation*—"Being a stay at home mom is the toughest work I've ever done. I want my husband and kids to know how hard I work even though I don't technically have a job."
- *Support*—"I need people around me who get me. Sometimes I feel like I've got to do everything alone, and it's hard. As a single mom, it helps so much when someone comes alongside of me and offers a helping hand and encouragement."
- *Money*—"If we had more money, we wouldn't have as much stress. It sure would solve a lot of our problems."
- *Morning workouts* (You know I liked this answer.)—"That time spent in the morning is my 'me time,' it's how I work through my stress and have the energy to get through the day. I'm not a nice person without it."
- *Feeling loved*—"When my husband does the dishes because I'm too tired or my kids wrap their arms around me and squeeze me really tight, my heart smiles."

While these are great responses, they are also circumstantial. Your husband won't always appreciate you. You won't always feel supported by others. Money comes and money goes. You may get injured and not be able to workout for a few weeks. Sometimes the dishes will pile up, your husband will choose football over vacuuming, or your kids will be too embarrassed to be seen hugging you.

Do you see what I'm saying? We can't hitch our happiness to anything that varies from day to day. Our emotional state can disrupt our fitness goals, so we need to take our focus off of our feelings and place it on our "Why."

Rejoice in the Lord always; again I will say, rejoice.
—Philippians 4:4 ESV

The enemy wants us to be unhappy. He came to kill, steal, and destroy. If he can keep us down, we can't come alive in the purposes God has designed for us.

I'm not a naturally happy person. You know those people who are always smiling and who are always in a good mood? Well, honestly, that's just not me. I grew up with alcoholism and abuse in my family, so my natural tendency is to be negative. But God has helped me see past any pain in my childhood and to change my mind to be more positive about life.

Since I became a Christian, God has renewed me through the Word and changed my perspective. He has made me happy from the inside out. Spending time in the Word every day healed those old pains, taught me how to find forgiveness, and has shown me that how I started isn't how I will finish.

People are always looking for the secret to a happy life. The secret is that there is no secret. It's all our decision. We choose the life we want. Free will allows us to choose, but it can also be that foot that

We can make the right choices in the midst of our wrong feelings; it's all about changing our perspectives from "have to" to "able to."

keeps tripping us. Bad attitudes and self-justification take us to the same place, which is nowhere near the life we want. But we can make the right choices in the midst of our wrong feelings; it's all about changing our perspectives from "have to" to "able to."

The Happy-Healthy Connection

Our emotions are directly related to our health. If we're committed to getting healthy but misery eats away at us on the inside, then we're tripping over ourselves. What's the first thing we do when we're stressed or depressed? We turn to our vices. Food is the most popular way women deal with their emotions. And, though eating through a bag of chips or shoving chocolate down our throats may comfort and take the edge off for a moment, these practices are not solutions. We need to address our negative emotions and deal with them through the Word, not food.

For you have been bought with a price: therefore glorify God in your body.
—1 Corinthians 6:20 NASB

We all have a God-shaped hole that makes us hungry for comfort, approval, achievement, and more. Often we try to fill that hole with these temporary securities either by excessive consumption and the feeling of releasing control or self-deprivation for the sake of feeling strong and in-control. Instead, we need to read what God says about the emotions we experience. A box of donuts might temporarily numb our pain, and resisting might make us feel unstoppable, but when we research what the Word says, we can move past our hurt and find happiness and health.

What's your happy-thief?

The first time my nervously-shaking hands touched the keyboard to write this book it was obvious my fearful thoughts were getting the best of me. *Who am I to write a book? What if it doesn't help anyone? What if I don't finish?* Fear (my happy-thief) had kept me from my goals before, but I wasn't going to allow it this time. I saved Isaiah 40:31, " Fear not for I am with you," on the home screen of my laptop to remind me to not let fear win.

I've battled with fear and doubt my entire life—fear that I wasn't good enough, fear of the unknown, and fear of not having control. This stemmed from growing up in an abusive home and made me very guarded and unsure of myself, but God changed me. I have my moments where the old tape recorder starts playing, but now I can spot the lies quickly and I'm armed with scriptures that speak the truth of who I am.

Whatever issues keep you from being happy are poisonous. These "happy-thieves" creep in and drain your energy and passion for life. They talk you into putting your emotions on the throne of your life and they excuse your behavior.

A happy-thief steals joy and can take different forms, such as:

- **Fear**
- **Unrealistically high expectations**
- **Bitterness**
- **Resentment**
- **Sadness**
- **Anger**
- **Jealousy**
- **Excuses**
- **Laziness**
- **Indifference**

Learning to find joy despite circumstantially negative emotions is a life lesson that only God can teach. Like the Israelites, we need to move past the shame or guilt of our failure and find joy in the knowledge that God is cheering us on and will help us every step of the way along our Faith Inspired Transformation. Just as it took minutes to impact my emotions and change my perspective after encountering the winning outlook of the incredible, older gentleman who survived a stroke, it only takes minutes in the Word of God to overcome our happy-thieves and find strength in the joy of the Lord.

LASTING JOY

We need to stop the cycle of feeling sad, mad, hurt, or even lonely and eating to numb our pain. Doing so makes us feel worse in the long run and gets us nowhere. Living out this health journey with God means we live in the light and not in darkness. We put Him on the throne and ask Him to take our hand and help navigate us through day-to-day life. Let's choose to desire the truth about ourselves and find contentment in Him and not in food.

You will keep in perfect peace all who trust in you, all whose thoughts are fixed on you!
—Isaiah 26:3 NLT

Content in Any State

I can do all things through Christ who strengthens me.
—Philippians 4:13 JUB

When I first became a Christian, Philippians 4:13 was one of my favorite verses. But, as I learned more about the apostle Paul's story in the Bible, I realized I had missed the depth of what this letter to the Philippians was saying.

As a man who often found himself imprisoned, who was shipwrecked at one point, and who was constantly moving from place to place and spreading the gospel, Paul knew how to get by with very little. He knew how to deal with going hungry because he was not always guaranteed a meal on his travels or while in prison, and he was fine suffering in need because he had lost everything during that fateful trip to Damascus (see Acts 9) and gained something far greater. In his writings, Paul points to Jesus Christ as his strength, the one giving him the ability to live through and endure any circumstance. In Him, Paul was content in any state.

Content in any state? Going hungry? Suffering need? I'll admit I'm not there. How about you?

We should be able to find contentment in any situation because we can do all things through Christ who strengthens us. Promotions, weight loss, and money won't satisfy. Their thrills are short lived before we move on and want something new. The desire for "more" is insatiable, and only God is enough to satisfy.

Think about the quick fixes you've tried, the no-carb diet, the low-fat diet, the juice fast, or even the exercise equipment you've wanted and bought. Did they mean anything to you after a few months? Did your fast-fix weight loss last? Did that state-of-the-art treadmill make you happy? Making God part of your journey to health is the only long-lasting solution. It's going to take work, but finding contentment in our Savior in any situation is the secret to being happy all the time.

Happy People Have Purpose

Whether we're called to be a stay-at-home mom, the CEO of a company, or to enjoy retirement, we all have a purpose. We are valuable and called to make an impact.

There is only one you, and that makes you very special. In our big world it's easy to feel invisible, but did you know you have a ministry? I bet when you think of the word *ministry* you picture a big church and its staff members, but God has called each of us to be his ambassadors—to represent Him in our daily lives to the world around us. In Him we all have the ability to teach and guide other people to become more like Christ; and, because we are all uniquely gifted, this looks different for everyone.

> **So Christ himself gave the apostles, the prophets, the evangelists, the pastors and teachers, to equip his people for works of service, so that the body of Christ may be built up.**
>
> **—Ephesians 4:11-12 NIV**

A few years ago, I randomly blurted out, "I'm writing a book!" The words just jumped out of my mouth before I could stop them. It was a secret I had kept for years, but I couldn't hold it in any longer. My heart was full of words to inspire women to live a healthy lifestyle in Christ. The only problem was that I hadn't actually written anything and I had no idea where to begin.

I imagine many women feel about their weight-loss goals the same way I did about writing a book to help them: unsure. Achieving any goals God has placed on our hearts is intimidating at first. Believe me, writing ten chapters of a book is as daunting a feat as losing thirty or so pounds. However, even when nothing in reality looks like the vision is achievable, if God has purposed it, there is no limit.

> **Now all glory to God, who is able, through his mighty power at work within us, to accomplish infinitely more than we might ask or think.**
>
> **—Ephesians 3:20 NLT**

If we are unhealthy and unhappy, we often lack the confidence and drive to pursue our purposes, but when we spend time strengthening ourselves from the inside out, we fight for the lives we want to lead and those purposes are revealed and fulfilled.

Don't make the mistake of thinking a perfect opportunity to fulfill your purpose will present itself. We must be willing to step out in faith and work to accomplish the tasks God has set aside for us to complete. Think of a time when you realized that you were perfectly equipped to accomplish a specific task. Did it seem as if you have been intentionally prepared for that task beforehand? Sometimes the greatest happiness we can experience is found after we finish a work that we clearly felt called to do.

I wrote this book in the most unconventional way: waiting in the pick-up line at my daughter's school, scribbling away at Starbucks between work appointments, and finding any other random time I could. My goal was thirty minutes a day, and that was really all the extra time I had.

Writing took everything in me. I had never written a book before, and it is a strenuous process requiring much discipline, but at this point in my life I am no stranger to self-discipline. After years of learning self-control and time management for the wrong reasons—living up to an ideal standard and garnering approval from the fitness world—God has turned those skills around for His purposes in my life, which include developing the F.I.T. Power Hour as a tool to get healthy with Him and writing *F.I.T.* as a resource and encouragement for women who want to experience the same internal and external transformation through the Word.

Committing half an hour a day to write a whole book doesn't sound like enough. And although the words kept coming, it rarely felt easy. I'll admit there were times it seemed too big a task and I felt completely unqualified. However, my perspective changed when my daughter

If God brought you to it, He can bring you through it.

gave me a little green frog she made in kindergarten. He's got long eyelashes and wears the acronym F.R.O.G. (Fully Rely On God) across his chest. He sits at my desk and reminds me every day that even when I feel incapable, God has equipped me and I am able.

Having a purpose and knowing God has granted it and prepared us for it brings such joy to our lives. It's the kind of lasting motivation we need to see lasting results. When our goals seem too big or even impossible, we need to remember that if God brought us to them, He can bring us through them.

Purpose for Change

Our God-given purposes should inspire us to be the best we can be in every part of our lives. That includes our health and fitness. When the Israelites learned from the prophet Ezra that they had been living apart from God's commands, they knew things had to change. They wanted to follow God once again, and for them it meant changing their lifestyle. The same is true today when it comes to honoring God with our health.

Honoring God with our time and our health provides a structure to our day that leads to a more productive and satisfying lifestyle. When we commit to the F.I.T. Power Hour—time with God, time with self, and time in exercise—we make spiritual, mental, and physical health our priority, which brings about a perspective shift. We see our lives through a greater purpose than just a race to looking great for summer vacation. The short-term thinking goes away and the dedication to a healthy life shines through.

Combining faith and fitness makes us over from the inside out. Consequently, it's a transformation that shows up in every aspect of our lives. When we're truly happy and feeling great about our health and our lives, we are beacons of hope for others who might be struggling.

Let your light so shine before men, that they may see your good works, and glorify your Father which is in Heaven.

—Matthew 5:16 KJV

People often believe they will be happy if they lose a few extra pounds, but the truth is that they could lose the weight and still be unsatisfied with their lives. When we believe happiness will come from gaining something that requires no change, we need to adjust our perspectives back to Paul's and believe that we can be content in any state as long as our eyes remain fixed on God.

We must keep our perspectives in check. There are seasons in life that are tough, but we can't allow ourselves to get away from spiritually training our inner selves to be strong and to keep going—fighting the good fight in faith. God gives our lives purpose, and when we live out those purposes to the best of our ability, we are truly made happy.

If you can't figure out your purpose, figure out your passion. For your passion will lead you right into your purpose.

—Bishop T.D. Jakes

If you believe in Christ, you have every reason to be happy. It's difficult when we let negative emotions cloud our views, but a change in perspective is all it takes to see God at work in our lives.

Casting down imaginations, and every high thing that exalteth itself against the knowledge of God, and bringing into captivity every thought to the obedience of Christ.

—2 Corinthians 10:5 KJV

GET F.I.T.

Therefore, since we are surrounded by such a huge crowd of witnesses to the life of faith, let us strip off every weight that slows us down, especially the sin that so easily trips us up. And let us run with endurance the race God has set before us.

—Hebrews 12:1 NLT

Although we have emotions, they shouldn't have us. In order to be happy, we need to change our perspective, put God on the throne of our lives, we need to be able to be content in any state, and we need to walk in the purpose He has created for us. The purposes God gives us should inspire us toward health in order to represent Him to the best of our ability.

Reflection Questions:

- Consider the 81-year-old man I met on my morning run. When was a time you experienced an eye-opening change in perspective?

____

____

____

- What is your happy-thief? How will you get it to stop stealing your joy?

____

____

____

Incorporate the following strategies into your life and experience a change of perspective that will draw you closer to Him and fill you with the strength and joy to continue moving forward in your Faith Inspired Transformation.

GET F.I.T.

Strategy #1: Identify and manage stress. Stress causes us to focus only on our circumstances and ourselves. It is a negative emotion that needs to be replaced with a positive perspective. Prayer, journaling, and good talks with a close friend are all effective ways to deal with stress. (However, if the stress you're feeling is unbearable, seek medical help.)

Strategy #2: Know your purpose and priorities. When we are organized and living intentionally with a plan, we interpret our lives differently. Life is no longer happening to us, we are being prepared for a purpose and work hard to be the best we can be for that purpose.

Let's get your day priority-driven.

- Have a clear plan of what you need to accomplish daily.
- Have a method of organizing yourself and your time.
- Manage known distractions and time stealers.
- Give yourself a ten-minute margin—leave earlier, get up earlier, and prepare the night before.
- If you're not living in your purpose, start taking your life in that direction with prayer.

Strategy #3: Keep a gratitude journal. Choice is powerful, so choose to focus on what you're grateful for instead of on all the things you want. Don't let your thoughts constantly drift to the future or the past—putting off health for tomorrow or believing the health you used to have is now unobtainable.

Strategy #4: Schedule fun today and every day on purpose. Laugh, smile, and have fun by doing something you love, even if it's only for ten minutes a day. Go play outside with your kids, put on your favorite music and dance, plan a date night with your husband, or go have coffee with a friend. The dishes, work, and to-do lists will still be there when you're done.

GET F.I.T.

Strategy #5: Give back. Giving back might be as simple as cleaning out your closet and donating toys and clothes to charity or supporting a cause by taking part in a heart walk or a breast cancer run. Getting involved in a cause offers the opportunity to give back and get healthier, a double blessing!

> **Give, and you will receive. Your gift will return to you in full—pressed down, shaken together to make room for more, running over, and poured into your lap. The amount you give will determine the amount you get back.**
>
> **—Luke 6:38 NLT**

Strategy #6: Write a "Dear God, I Give You..." letter. What can you give God today? Trade your bitterness for forgiveness, your resentment for peace, your hurt for healing, and your disappointment for blessing. I know this is easier said than done, but you're never going to be happy holding onto your same old struggles.

> **You were bought at a price; do not become slaves of human beings.**
>
> **—1 Corinthians 7:23 NIV**

My father and I had a horrible time growing up. When he had a stroke, I knew I needed to forgive him – for me. God was able to heal those past hurts and restore our relationship. Now that he's gone, I'm so grateful that God spoke to my heart and showed me that I needed to put the pain behind us. A life of regret is more painful than choosing to forgive someone now—regardless of their actions.

Joanna Weaver's quote, "Bitterness is like drinking poison and waiting for the other person to die," perfectly embodies what not forgiving someone does to us. Choose to let it go for you.

GET F.I.T.

Dear God,

I give you...

If the joy of the Lord is our strength, then happiness isn't material; it's a choice we make in those tough moments to see Him working in our circumstances rather than focusing on our problems.

STEP NINE | OVERCOME SETBACKS

Stick to Your F.A.I.T.H. Goals

I keep my eyes always on the LORD. With him at my right hand, I will not be shaken.

—Psalm 16:8 NIV

What makes F.I.T. different from other programs is the daily commitment to keep our eyes fixed on God. The time spent in our daily F.I.T. Power Hour is meant, first and foremost, to help us grow in our faith. From that faith comes the desire and the strength to honor Him with healthy choices in other areas of our lives. When we get away from our time with Him, the cares of the world take over. For this reason, we must continue to go to the Word and not the world when setbacks cause us to swerve off course.

Okay, I know you're wondering, *How does this help me when I stand on my scale and I'm miserable about my weight or when I'm eating right and working out and I don't see any results? How do I keep going in those moments?* My answer is that we do it one day at a time in faith. I know this can seem impossible. I know every mistake feels like the end of the road. I've been there, and I know how painfully frustrating and hopeless it may feel. Transforming your health is difficult, but you're not alone. There is a process to getting healthy, and it takes time. You can't rush it. This is why faith makes all the difference.

If you aren't losing as much weight as you want, you are gaining weight, you've hit a plateau, you are tired of eating only God-made foods, or if your routine is off due to traveling, then you have encountered one of the many setbacks we all face from time to time.

When it appears you have hit a roadblock:

- Acknowledge the issue. Until you face the problem, nothing happens. Why has your progress stopped? Objectively evaluate your commitment. Did you get bored with what you were eating or with your workouts? Remember simple changes such as new recipes or group classes can pull you out of a rut.
- Journal how you feel about it. Take the time to acknowledge how you're feeling because avoidance will not get you back on track. We all mess up, get sick, have bad days, and sometimes don't feel like working out or eating right, but that doesn't mean we give up on our health goals.
- Remind yourself *why* you want to get healthy. Stir yourself up, make your "Why" relational, medical, or spiritual. If your "Why" is your children, the temptation to order a bucket of fried chicken or skip a workout should lose its appeal when you think about being a good role model for them.
- Recommit to your F.A.I.T.H. goals and to your F.I.T. Power Hour. Keep your goals in view. Write them on a sheet of paper and tape it somewhere, or make them your screen saver. Think about how much better you feel on the days when you get in your F.I.T. Power Hour than when you don't. Any time spent with God, on your health, and checking in with yourself is better than none at all.
- Pray for discernment and strength to keep moving forward. You may feel discouraged and want to quit when you don't see progress, but this is when you need to have faith that every good choice you make is adding up to results. Getting healthy is a process, so be faithful to your F.I.T. Power Hour and God will

give you all you need to stay the course.

- Don't just focus on the negatives; look at how far you've come. If you chose God-made, healthful foods all day but had a cookie for dessert, that doesn't mean today wasn't a good day. If you worked out three days this week instead of five, hooray for the three workouts you got in! Balance out the checklist in your mind with what you do right, and refrain from focusing on the things you don't do perfectly.

To stay the course it's important that we address some of these roadblocks that might spring up along our fitness journey and discuss ways to overcome them in order to move forward one day at a time.

IF YOU'RE NOT LOSING WEIGHT

In the book of Exodus, Moses led God's people through the wilderness for forty years before they were able to settle in a land he had prepared for them. Along the way they lost faith and forgot the promise God had given them of a better life. All the while, God was pleading with them to trust Him and keep walking in faith.

Just as it took time for God's people to reach the Promised Land, it takes time to reach our health goals, and we must remain patient and faithful in the process. As you journey on toward a good lifestyle God has promised to give you, don't become like the people of the Exodus. Don't get frustrated and discouraged because you're not seeing results, eat a bunch of garbage, and set yourself back even more. Be consistent, keep going, and you will see results. Expect slow and steady progress and know that there's nothing wrong with small beginnings.

Do not despise these small beginnings, for the Lord rejoices to see the work begin.

—Zechariah 4:10 NLT

Don't Trust ONLY the Scale

When you first begin an exercise program, be aware that the scale is not telling the whole story. Muscles are about eighty percent water, and when you put a lot of stress on them, they hold on to water in order to heal. This is temporary and your body will acclimate, so do not take it as a sign that working out is not working for you.

Another thing to consider is that muscle takes up a quarter of the space as fat. When I went through my transformation, my weight loss wasn't drastically different according to the scale, but my waist lost five inches and I went down four sizes.

Exercise and muscle gain redesigns our bodies. The scale doesn't account for changes in composition. You may gain muscle and lose fat and actually wear a smaller clothing size, but the scale may say you weigh more. Get on the scale as frequently as you need to, but never let it be the only measurement you take. Measuring tapes, fat calibers, before and after pictures, and even your favorite jeans are better ways to track progress.

Keep in mind the fact that you're a woman and the number on the scale will fluctuate with your monthly cycle. If you feel puffy and bloated on a regular basis, you are probably struggling with water weight. Also, bloating is actually caused by not drinking enough water because when your body isn't getting enough water it won't release the little that it has. So, make sure you're adequately hydrated, taking in a minimum of eight glasses of water each day.

If the scale makes you miserable, remember the number is not your report card. It doesn't define whether you are a success or a failure; it's just a number—that's it! The scale made me miserable for years. After exercising all week and eating healthy, God-made foods, I would wake up feeling great and would step on the scale only to see a number that made a tidal wave of self-loathing wash over me. *Ugh!* I got over this by weighing myself every day in order to understand how weight fluctuates, and now I rarely weigh myself at all.

Realize that weight is just a number, so develop a healthy relationship with the scale. It's very liberating.

Finally, refrain from comparing what you weigh to what the magazines say someone else weighs because there is a good chance they aren't telling the truth. Unfortunately, people have been lying about their weight for decades. It's sad and perpetuates the feeling of failure among women who buy into the lies, so don't be one of those women who define themselves solely by a magazine image or a number on the scale.

Weight is just a number, so develop a healthy relationship with the scale.

Consider Your Method of Weight Loss

While I encourage you not to focus only on your weight, it should still give you some indication of progress. Therefore, if you are trying to lose weight and not seeing your desired results, consider reevaluating your methods. Even if you eat considerably less food than normal, you still might not reach your fitness goals. It all depends on your methods.

For instance, chronic dieting causes muscle loss, which raises body fat. This makes it harder and harder to lose weight because your body actually becomes less metabolically active. Furthermore, counting calories is a common tool for weight loss but, as I mentioned earlier, not all calories are created equally, so the source of the calories is the real issue, not necessarily the amount you are consuming.

Overhearing many conversations at the gym, I once heard a girl tell her friend that it was time to burn off the donuts they had eaten earlier that morning. While our bodies are going to burn calories when we work out, the way our bodies look will be greatly affected by the type of calories we take in before and after exercising. You can't trade time spent on the treadmill for the number of donuts you've consumed because your body is much more complex than that. In short, you can't just eliminate the junk you put into your body by exercising more. Don't try to cheat the system.

F.I.T. is all about finding balance in your health *and* fitness. To reap the benefits of one, we must be mindful of the other. Furthermore, eating processed foods and doing solely cardio will raise your body fat percentage.

In other words, don't just run every day and never perform any other sort of strength training. Performing long periods of slow cardio cause you to burn muscle, which decreases your metabolism. The worry I encounter most from women is that resistance training will make them big and bulky, but this is a myth. Balance cardio with strength training or body weight training to maintain lean-muscle mass (the calorie burner) and feed your body God-made foods.

Beat the Plateau

If you've committed to your health but you're not seeing any results, you may have hit a plateau. But don't worry! There are ways to get past it if you understand why it's occurring.

Below are problems that might be causing you to plateau and the corresponding solutions to help you get past it.

Problem: You're not eating enough. Excessively restricting calories causes your metabolism to slow down and, therefore, you burn fewer calories.
Solution: Make sure you're eating three to five healthy meals a day and getting in your strength training to maintain your lean muscle mass, the calorie burner.

Problem: You've gained muscle mass, but you're not seeing weight loss on the scale.
Solution: Don't rely on scale weight as your only measurement. Your lean body weight is increasing and your body fat is decreasing.

Problem: You're in a rut doing the same workout. The human body is the master of adaptation—same old exercises and cardio machine makes the same old body.
Solution: Your muscles have to work much harder when you do something new, so keep your body guessing by switching up your workouts. High intensity interval training (HIIT), TRX, or anything you've never done before are all great ways to shock your body and get it past a plateau.

Problem: You eat great all week, but you eat whatever you want on the weekends. Basically, you're gaining and losing the same few pounds and never making any progress.
Solution: Enjoy one or two meals of whatever you want on the weekend, but don't throw your health goals out the window. Have a barbeque, grill meat and veggies and get active with your friends and family. No matter what type of meal you're eating, always remember to implement the 5 Ps.

IF YOU'RE TIRED OF GOD-MADE FOODS

The very first time I competed in a fitness competition, I was immersed in the learning process of how to eat right. I thought the best thing to do was find out what everyone else was doing. Learning that the majority of women ate lean protein and veggies every three hours, six times a day, was grueling. And, although I was eating God-made foods, there was no way I could live on that menu.

God-made eating isn't dieting, and it isn't boring; it's our habits that lead us to the same boring food choices.

Food boredom can ruin your desire to eat healthfully, but it doesn't have to be that way. New recipes and restaurants are an easy way to relieve food monotony, and healthy versions of dishes, such as homemade lasagna, chicken fingers, pizza, and burgers, dispel the typical suffering that is implied with healthy eating.

God-made eating isn't dieting, and it isn't boring; it's our habits that lead us to the same boring food choices. Get out of your food rut by mixing things up and making food fun. Try new recipes, experiment with different spices, and even make your own salad dressings and marinades to capture your favorite flavors. Eating should be enjoyable, and your food should taste good if you're going to maintain a healthy lifestyle.

IF YOU'RE TRAVELING

Working for an outside sales company made my client Julie profess to being in the worst shape of her life. Spending weeks at a time away from home and then being on the road all day made healthful eating and consistent exercise a challenge. Confessing that she ate only one large meal a day and rarely exercised made Julie feel horrible. More than losing weight, she just wanted to feel good again.

Like many other women, Julie had a hard time managing her health and fitness when her routine was mixed up with traveling. Don't we find it difficult to keep up with our daily commitments when our days look different than normal? In such instances, especially when it comes to traveling, I think it's best to have a game plan laid out before you ever hit the road.

Examples of ways to plan ahead when traveling are as follows:

- Keep a healthy snack or protein shake in your purse. This is as simple as a pack of almonds or carrot sticks or an individual protein shake packet.

- If you work from your car or travel frequently, invest in an insulated food carrier. Being prepared and packing leftovers, your favorite drinks, and plenty of snacks and shakes to keep food fresh and on hand will make staying healthy simple.
- Refrain from the free-for-all mentality vacations can cause you to have about food. When I'm traveling I have a shake for breakfast (Isagenix, Isalean shakes are my go-to because of their dedication to the highest quality ingredients, plus they taste great!), but you could also keep raw nuts, veggies, and fruit with you and skip the all-you-can-eat buffet at the hotel.
- When ordering at a restaurant, choose grilled meats and veggies or healthy salads with a choice of one or two toppings (nuts, raisins, dressing, croutons, cheese, or avocado) but not all of them, as that is how a salad ends up having more calories than a small pizza. Ask to leave off extra butter or oils used for meat and vegetable preparation. Many restaurants now offer smaller portions or healthy choice menus. Look for these and be mindful of portion sizes. If there are no smaller portions or healthy menu options, order a to-go box and pack up half of your entrée as soon as your meal arrives. This is a great way to save money and calories.
- When you check-in to a hotel, ask where the local grocery store is and request a mini fridge in your room. Stock it with healthy options.
- Stay active. Find a place to enjoy the outdoors—take scenic walks and enjoy a new jogging trail.
- Have a go-to workout for your hotel room, in case there's no gym and if it's snowing or raining outside, by bringing your laptop and your fitness DVDs or by going to YouTube and

choosing a new workout every day.

- Have excuse-proof equipment for "on the go." Some of my favorites (all of which can be purchased online or at a sports store) include:
    - Gliders—two little discs (you can substitute paper plates or socks on a tile floor) that enable you to do a variety of low impact cardio—running, mountain climbers, and upper body swimming exercises—that will make you more tired than sprinting. They pack easily, are great if you have any pain doing high impact cardio, and they enable you to work out in a very small area.
    - Resistance bands
    - Therabands
    - Jump ropes
    - TRX suspension straps
    - An inflatable exercise ball
- Stick to a consistent sleep schedule by going to bed and getting up at the same time every day. Aim for seven to eight hours of sleep per night for optimal health.

Sharing these tips with Julie, she found that having the insulated food carrier and learning how to order from a restaurant menu provided healthy options she hadn't considered before. She now enjoys her home-cooked meals from the front seat of her car. And, as an extra bonus, she also saves money. Having a passion for running, Julie now gets her run in before the day begins. Instead of making excuses to skip a workout when traveling, she googles places to run before she arrives at her destination.

A few simple changes changed everything for Julie, and they can do the same for you. Don't let setbacks hold you down any longer. Stay committed and get creative as you create your own excuse-proof game plan.

GET F.I.T.

When conquering anything new, there are bound to be a few roadblocks. We must prepare ourselves to get back up after a fall, rely on God (our rock) through scripture and prayer, and assess our weaknesses to discover ways to keep them from getting us down in the future.

It is vital that we continue to seek God's best for our health when we:

- aren't losing weight;
- hit a plateau;
- grow tired of eating God-made foods; or
- travel.

If you've fallen off the wagon, stopped losing weight, or you're bored with God-made foods, then you might be facing a setback to your Faith Inspired Transformation. Follow the strategies below to find success in the face of a potential setback, and stick to your F.A.I.T.H. goals.

Strategy #1: Be proactive. Acknowledge what you're feeling and why it's happening. When you put off getting healthy or hit the pause button on your health goals, the only person you're hurting is yourself. Revisit your "Why" and your F.A.I.T.H. goals, and rededicate your health to God. Make your next health decision a good one.

Strategy #2: Be committed. When weight loss stalls, evaluate your commitment and your methods. Are you showing up for your F.I.T. Power Hour? Are you following the 5 Ps? Could weekends be derailing your progress? Getting healthy requires change and commitment.

Strategy #3: Be prepared. Plan for health success by keeping snacks in your purse, packing leftovers for lunch, and learning new recipes and exercises as often as you can. In doing so you will save yourself from food boredom and weight loss plateaus.

Strategy #4: Enjoy an occasional treat. F.I.T. is not a diet, and we're doing real life together. So, occasionally enjoy a burger, but skip the fries and say yes to steamed veggies or a salad with dressing on the side, or split an entrée with your husband, child, or friend. Don't deprive yourself of the foods you enjoy, just remember to practice self-control when you have an occasional treat.

Strategy #5: Have faith! Always turn to God when you're ready to quit. Ask Him to invigorate your spirit and help you believe that every good decision you're making is taking you a step closer to your health goals.

STEP TEN | CELEBRATE EVERY VICTORY

Become a New You in Him

Ask, and it will be given to you; seek, and you will find; knock, and it will be opened to you.
—Matthew 7:7 ESV

One day Lynn, a lovely lady from church, shared with me her humorous view of health and fitness. With a big smile, she referred to a healthy lifestyle as a monster that wanted to take away everything she loved—the food that she would have to give up on a diet and the comfort of her own home she would give up to go to a gym.

We both laughed!

Understanding that she related getting healthy with deprivation and discomfort, I formulated a game plan that focused on what she loved doing. In learning more about Lynn, I discovered she had a passion for cooking and that she loved to dance. So, meeting with her once a week, I gave Lynn a list of simple fixes, such as trading sugar for stevia, baking with unsweetened applesauce rather than butter or oils, and trying three smaller meals and a snack versus two large meals a day. Because she loved to dance, I suggested working out to a Zumba video and thought that she would enjoy this type of workout enough to stick with it, especially since she could do it in the privacy of her own home.

These F.I.T ideas, though simple, proved to be effective in creating a lasting change for Lynn. A year later, those little changes have evolved into a lifestyle transformation for her. And, as Lynn is now a Zumba instructor, she is changing other people's lives as well.

Celebrate Small Wins

People think success comes at a particular point in time—earning a degree, making a down payment on a beautiful home, or even picking a winning lottery ticket. But when it comes to changing our health, success is all about the daily win because the momentum of small victories sets our motivation on fire. As Charles Duhigg explains with the Theory of Small Wins in his book, *The Power of Habit*, "Small wins fuel transformative changes by leveraging tiny advantages into patterns that convince people that bigger achievements are within reach."[13] These little, faithful wins in our daily decisions remind us that we are able.

It's the "No, I'll have an iced green tea, not a latte," it's the extra push-up when you want to quit, and it's the choice to take the stairs instead of the escalator that makes the difference. Create small wins each day.

- **Choose water over soda at dinner.**
- **Eat oatmeal instead of a pastry for breakfast.**
- **Split your typically larger lunch into two smaller meals.**
- **Order a side salad instead of fries or chips**
- **Choose raw veggies and hummus for a snack instead of a candy bar.**
- **Go for a run first thing in the morning.**
- **Lift five pounds more than you normally do in the weight room.**

Because we have a tendency to catalog the things we don't do well, we need to retrain our brains to see the success in ourselves. Rather than thinking about what we have done wrong, let's focus on everything we have done right, we are doing right, and we will begin to do right.

This is how we own our part in our faith and fitness journeys:

- **ask (pray)**
- **seek (work)**
- **keep knocking (persevere)**

Sometimes our daily win isn't with food or fitness; sometimes it's a faith challenge, and we know the only way we can do this is in Him. As we continue to see small victories in our faith and fitness, we grow in our Godfidence. And, because we are more than our bodies, it doesn't end there. God does not want us to settle for small victories; he wants to make us more than conquerors.

Faith means we believe without seeing proof. It means we do the hard stuff, such as making the right choices, even when we don't see immediate results, and especially when we'd rather make excuses. So, be sure to acknowledge your small wins. Every victory is worth celebrating, no matter how small.

Celebrate your F.I.T. victories with something other than food. Some ideas include:

- visiting an art show, gallery, or a local museum,
- going to the movies with a friend,
- doing something on your bucket list,
- having your hair done (and maybe learning a few tricks from your stylist),
- inviting friends over,
- buying a special candle and enjoying a long bath with a great book,
- pampering yourself with a massage,
- buying yourself a new outfit,
- treating yourself to a manicure and pedicure, and
- having a professional give you a makeover (learn quick tips on makeup from the best).

Celebrate Your Courage to Persist

I am the vine, you are the branches; he who abides in Me and I in him, he bears much fruit, for apart from Me you can do nothing.

—John 15:5 NASB

Driving to Tucson on a chilly February morning, the sky was beautiful shades of pink, orange, and purple as the sun was barely peeking over the mountains. I was alone on the road and excited about speaking at a women's church group. The topic was a great one: how to have a physically, emotionally and spiritually healthy heart.

Despite my excitement, I found myself really struggling. This talk was going to be harder than others because this church was where my father's funeral services had been held, and I hadn't been there since. It was about a two-hour drive, so I had a lot of time to fight back the tears. I didn't want to show up looking like a mess with mascara running down my face.

Determined to do my best for these ladies, I started flipping through the radio stations, and I landed on Sara Bareilles' song "Brave." It was exactly what I needed to hear. (Isn't God's timing perfect?) Feeling so weak, I knew I needed to put on my Godfidence and find the courage to keep going. This is how we own our part in our faith and fitness journeys: ask (pray), seek (work), and keep knocking (persevere).

Sometimes we need to suck it up in the spirit and get to work. We have to show up, even when it's hard, really hard. This is true in our fitness, in our health, and in our daily lives. And, when we are brave enough to turn our eyes to God and away from our problems, and even our excuses, and find the strength to become the women He has made us to be, you better believe that is something worth celebrating.

So, let's be brave. Let's be brave enough to stick to our commitments, brave enough to believe in ourselves, and brave enough to trust that God is working all things together for good.

A brave woman is one who:

B – Believes in faith that God answers bold prayers.
R – Rejoices as the Lord revives her according to His Word.
A – Abides in Him and takes action.
V – Vanquishes her foes (negative thoughts, unhealthy foods, laziness, etc.).
E – Endures all things and keeps her eyes focused on God's eternal purposes.

Believing, rejoicing, and abiding in God and vanquishing our foes and enduring all things with His help are the ways in which we become brave. We can do these things because He is with us always. However, apart from Him we can do nothing. That's why this journey is about taking control of our bodies and then handing that control right back to God to find lasting health. Thankfully, He doesn't make us do it on our own, and we show our courage when we release that control and trust that He is the one who changes everything.

God changes everything!

Celebrate the Impossible

Jesus replied, "The things that are impossible for people are possible for God."
—Luke 18:27 ISV

When we look back over our lives, we often see where God was working. But it can be difficult to see Him at work when we're in the middle of something challenging. But, nevertheless, He *is* there enabling us to survive issues we never thought our hearts could handle.

I wanted so badly to do another fitness competition after my daughter was born, but by that time I turned forty and had become lax in my fitness and eating habits—the idea was laughable. I was happy with my life, and there wasn't any particular reason I wanted to get on stage with a bunch of eighteen-year-old Olympic gymnasts, I just missed competing. For whatever reason, the desire to push my body beyond its limits was a part of myself that I couldn't deny any longer.

So, as I gently pushed my eighteen-month-old daughter on the swings one warm summer evening, I told my husband that I wanted to compete in the Fox Sports Ms. Fitness USA competition. It was almost embarrassing to say, but my sweet husband just smiled and said, "Okay!"

It had been about seven years since I had won the ESPN Fitness America competition. I was older and still hadn't lost all of the weight gained during my pregnancy. Needless to say, the training I subjected myself to for Ms. Fitness was grueling, at times unbearably so. I figured I didn't stand a chance and questioned why I was even bothering to work so hard, but this small voice inside of me said to keep going.

When I was finally standing on the Ms. Fitness USA stage, I didn't care if I won or lost. I looked around and felt so blessed to be in the company of such talented women, knowing that I had already won the greatest prize along my life's journey: a lifelong relationship with God. I remembered the overweight, unhappy person I had once been and felt so grateful for the love He had continuously poured into my life. Winning or losing or placing anywhere in between didn't matter in that moment because I was already celebrating God's victory over the impossible in my life.

When it was announced that I had won the fitness routine portion of the competition and placed second overall, I took it as reminder from God that it's never too late, and it became clear to me that He had prepared me for this victory, at age forty, for a very specific purpose. It wasn't so that I could boast about myself or find confidence that might have been lost. No, I believe God put me on that stage to show me that He could and because I knew I couldn't have gotten there without Him.

God has you right where you are, wherever you are, for a specific purpose as well. Maybe it's not on the stage of a fitness competition, maybe it's somewhere you really would rather not be. No matter where you are, the fact remains that God is right there with you, He is taking you where He wants you to go, and the word *impossible* is not in his vocabulary. Don't focus your efforts on achieving health and fitness in your own strength—there will never be enough of it. Bring it to God, all that you have, and let Him show you what's really possible.

God has you right where you are, wherever you are, for a specific purpose.

Celebrate You

> **Not that I have already obtained this or am already perfect, but I press on to make it my own, because Christ Jesus has made me his own. Brothers, I do not consider that I have made it my own. But one thing I do: forgetting what lies behind and straining forward to what lies ahead, I press on toward the goal for the prize of the upward call of God in Christ Jesus.**
>
> **—Philippians 3:12-14 ESV**

Maybe you're reading this book and you're not a Christian or you've lost your faith. Even if you don't buy into this now, think about whether or not focusing on (and maybe even achieving) a certain look ever gave you the satisfaction you wanted. I know it was never enough for me. Choosing my identity in Christ over my identity as a fitness model, businesswoman, mother, wife, or anything else is what transformed me. It was my point of transformation in faith and in my health and fitness.

I believe God wants you to have a fulfilled life. Let Him be your motivation. Get in the Word, and let it make you strong and healthy from the inside out.

"Press on." "Keep going." "Don't stop." "Quitting is not an option." We see these motivational phrases applied to every human goal. As Christians, our goal is to have the right motives and to please God in everything we do. He has a plan and a purpose that only we can carry out, so we can't give up on ourselves. God has made us each unique and has given us desires and preferences and skills that will help us maintain a healthy lifestyle that honors Him. Our challenge is to press on when we want to give up and to celebrate the people He is making each of us into.

> **So do not throw away your confidence; it will be richly rewarded. You need to persevere so that when you have done the will of God, you will receive what he has promised.**
>
> **—Hebrews 10:35-36 NIV**

You are strong and capable. Celebrate your strength and your ability to continue on this journey, and don't worry about tomorrow. Og Mandino's "I will persist until I succeed" from *The Greatest Salesman in the World* captures this very idea. Read it and remember that, "in truth, one step at a time is not too difficult."

I Will Persist Until I Succeed

The prizes of life are at the end of each journey, not near the beginning; and it is not given to me to know how many steps are necessary in order to reach my goal. Failure I may still encounter at the thousandth step, yet success hides behind the next bend in the road. Never will I know how close it lies unless I turn the corner.

Always will I take another step. If that is of no avail I will take another, and yet another. In truth, one step at a time is not too difficult.

I will persist until I succeed.[14]

God is asking you to take the next step with Him. He knows you, loves you, and is preparing a way for you. You can reach your health and fitness goals, but just remember that it's not the destination which holds the lasting reward; our reward is found in the relationship we build with Him every step of the way.

F.I.T. FOR VICTORY

Combining our faith with our fitness means we are done with the finish-line mentality. We are in it for the marathon of life. We walk our health out daily with God as our partner, and He changes us to become who we are meant to be in Christ. He refines us and renews our minds to see our world through His Word. Growing in the character and nature of God is what we can expect from our F.I.T. Power Hour, and the physical changes that come from exercise and enjoying God-made foods are just added benefits.

F.I.T. doesn't have a tricky marketing scheme. There isn't a restrictive plan or any reliance on a product. We rely in faith on God's promises, we eat God-made foods, and we bring our bodies under our control through Him.

God promises that, if you will seek Him, you will find Him if you seek Him with all your heart and with all your soul. The Lord is near to all who call upon Him, to all who call upon Him in truth. Draw near to God and He will draw near to you.

God is not a supplement to our life, and He isn't a part of the F.I.T. program; He is the heart of the matter. He is our focus, and He gives us the ability to walk in self-control. That is the freedom we are looking for, isn't it? It's a freedom that we won't find in a diet that may or may not give us a beach body for one week. It's a lifelong commitment that never goes unreturned. It's something that should be celebrated every step of the way because He is taking every step with us.

Fight for what you want in this life. A Faith Inspired Transformation means you can't live with old habits and see new results. Keep believing and rejoicing with every step forward, as you become a new you in Him.

Blessed is she who has believed that the Lord would fulfill his promises to her!

—Luke 1:45 NIV

GET F.I.T.

Our daily choices make all the difference, so celebrate when you make the right ones. Remember, no victory is too small. This is not about perfection. Every step forward is progress, and God is right there cheering you along. Continue to seek Him in your Faith Inspired Transformation and rejoice as you become a new you in Him.

Reflection Questions:

- What small win did you create for yourself today?

  ____

- How will you choose to celebrate your health victories?

  ____

- What hardship have you overcome? If you're in the middle of one right now, how do you think God can use it to make you stronger?

  ____

  ____

- How will combining your faith with your fitness change your approach to eating, exercising and the way you think about health?

  ____

  ____

Thank you for taking this journey with me. I want you to know I am here for you and I am praying for you every step of the way. My website is dedicated to providing you with the tools, resources, and support necessary to help you on your Faith Inspired Transformation. Please check it out, and feel free to offer your thoughts, ask questions, and even share your F.I.T. Story. I would love to hear from you.

—Kim

GET F.I.T.

10 Steps to F.I.T.

1. **Stop Dieting: Get Healthy For Good with God**—This is where we identify the failures of quick-fix dieting and agree to embark on the Faith Inspired Transformation.
2. **Renew Your Mind: See Yourself Through the Word and Not the World**—This is where we turn our focus from changing our bodies to changing our lifestyle according to God's Word.
3. **Commit to the F.I.T. Power Hour: Practice Spiritual, Mental, and Physical Fitness**—This is a daily commitment to spend time in the Word of God, time alone and in prayer, and time exercising.
4. **Dress Yourself with Strength: Make Your Arms Strong and Put on "Godfidence"**—This is where we learn about different forms of exercise and ask God to help us become physically strong.
5. **Set F.A.I.T.H. Goals: Plan For Success**—These are faith-filled, accountable, inspirational, timely, and healthy goals and strategies we set for ourselves as we strive to get healthy, happy, and fit God's way.
6. **Eat God-made, Not Man-made Foods: Make Healthy Easy**—Here we learn simple ways to portion out and enjoy healthful meals using the God-made Hand Chart and choosing God-made foods.
7. **Choose Self-Control: Find Lasting Motivation and Implement the 5 Ps**—By finding motivation that lasts (basing it in something relational, medical, or spiritual) and implementing the 5 Ps (Pause, Pray, Portion, Practice, Plan), we learn to practice self-control.
8. **Change Your Perspective: Find Joy in Every Situation**—In this step we see changing our health and fitness as something we are able to do rather than something we have to do.
9. **Overcome Setbacks: Get a F.A.I.T.H. Lift**—Here we remember our F.A.I.T.H. goals to deal with setbacks and proactively strategize ways to keep exercising regularly and eating God-made foods even when our circumstances change.
10. **Celebrate Every Victory: Become a New You in Him**—Finally, we celebrate the work we have been doing and every victory we have encountered, no matter how small it may seem.

NOTES

Step 1: "Stop Dieting": Get Healthy For Good With God

1. ABC News Staff, "100 Million Dieters, $20 Billion: The Weight-Loss Industry by the Numbers," Containing information from John LaRosa of MarketData; National Weight Control Registry; American Society for Metabolic and Bariatric Surgery; Jo Piazza, author of *Celebrity Inc.: How Famous People Make Money*, May 8, 2012. http://abcnews.go.com/Health/100-million-dieters-20-billion-weight-loss- industry/story?id=16297197

2. National Center for Health Statistics.Health, United States, 2013: With Special Feature on Prescription Drugs. Hyattsville, MD. 2014. http://www.cdc.gov/nchs/data/hus/hus13.pdf#064

Step 2: "Renew Your Mind": See Yourself Through the Word, Not the World

3. Daniel G. Amen, M.D., "ANT Therapy: How to Develop Your Own Internal Anteater to Eradicate Automatic Negative Thoughts." The American Holistic Health Association self-help article. http://ahha.org/articles.asp?Id=100

Step 3: "Commit to the F.I.T. Power Hour": Practice Spiritual, Mental, and Physical Fitness

4. Dr. Stephen R. Covey, "The Big Rocks of Life." http://www.apleseeds.org/Big-Rocks_Covey.htm

Step 4: "Dress Yourself With Strength": Put on "Godfidence"

5. Division of Nutrition, "Physical Activity and Obesity," National Center for Chronic Disease Prevention and Health Promotion, February 16, 2011. http://www.cdc.gov/physicalactivity/everyone/health/.

*Figure 1 chart modified from: Cindy Brotherston, "Heart Rate Monitor: What for?...Which One?...and How Much?", The "Right" Intensity: Find Your Target Zone chart, December 1, 2014 (date accessed). www.busywomensfitness.com/heart-rate-monitor.html

*Figure 2 chart modified from: Jessica Wurtzebach, Castle Hill Fitness Blog, "Dispelling the 220-age Myth." Target heart rate zone chart. December 1, 2014 (date accessed). www.castlehillfitness.com/blog/2012/07/dispelling-the-220-age-myth/

6. American Heart Association, Get Healthy, Physical Activity, "Target Heart Rates." Instructions for checking heart rate. September 23, 2014. http://www.heart.org/HEARTORG/GettingHealthy/PhysicalActivity/FitnessBasics/Target-Heart-Rates_UCM_434341_Article.jsp

Step 6: "Eat God-made, Not Man-made": Make Healthy Easy

7. Dr. Stephen Sinatra's Heart MD Institute, Health Topics, Diabetes & Obesity, "Ultra-Processed Food and Obesity," May 9, 2011. http://www.heartmdinstitute.com/health-topics/diabetes-obesity/203-ultra-processed-food-obesity.

8. Martina M. Cartwright, Ph.D., R.D., "Three Reasons Dieters Should Eat More Protein," *Psychology Today*, July 25, 2013. http://www.psychologytoday.com/blog/food-thought/201307/three-reasons-dieters-should-eat-more-protein.

9. Brian Krans, "Sugar Is a 'Drug' and Here's How We're Addicted

Hooked," Healthline News, September 18, 2013. http://www.healthline.com/health-news/addiction-sugar-acts-like-drug-in-the-brain-and-could-lead-to-addiction-091813.

10. Karen Kaplan, "Can you eat only 6 teaspoons of sugar a day? The WHO wants you to try," *Los Angeles Times*, March 5, 2014. http://www.latimes.com/science/sciencenow/la-sci-sn-added-sugar-who-six-teaspoons-per-day-20140305-story.html

11. "Exercise Vs. Diet: The Truth About Weight Loss," Quote from Shawn M. Talbott, PhD, nutritional biochemist and former director of the University of Utah Nutrition Clinic. http://www.huffingtonpost.com/2014/04/30/exercise-vs-diet-for-weight-loss_n_5207271.html.

Step 7: "Choose Self-Control": Find Lasting Motivation and Implement the 5 Ps

12. Gretchen Voss, "When you lose weight—and gain it all back." Diet & nutrition on NBCNEWS.com, June 6, 2010. (Rodale Inc., 2012). http://www.nbcnews.com/id/36716808/ns/health-diet_and_nutrition/t/when-you-lose-weight-gain-it-all-back/#.VD_Yh75h2RZ

Step 10: "Celebrate Every Victory": Become A New You In Him

13. Charles Duhigg, *The Power of Habit*, trade paperback edition, Random House, New York, January 7, 2014.

14. Og Mandina, *The Greatest Salesman In the World,* "I will persist until I succeed," Bantam trade edition, Feb. 1985.

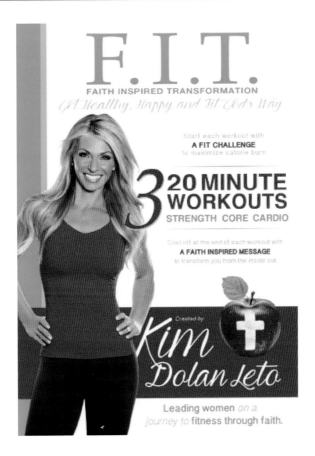